NO PICNIC

An Insider's Guide to Tickborne Illnesses

PJ Langhoff

No Picnic

An Insider's Guide to Tickborne Illnesses

Published by Allegory Press, LLC, Hustisford, WI, 53034
First Standard Edition
Printed in the United States of America

ISBN: 978-0-9833765-6-9
Library of Congress Control Number: 2013910943

For more information or for permissions, please contact the author at:
PJ Langhoff
c/o Allegory Press LLC
PO Box 444
Hustisford, WI 53034, USA
books@allegorypress.com

Downloadable booklet is available at: www.Allegorypress.com

See the other great books by this author at:
www.Allegorypress.com
www.Amazon.com
and other book sellers

Images are provided by the Centers for Disease Control (CDC) except as marked.
Typefaces are Papyrus and Times New Roman.

Printed in the United States of America

Table of Contents

Disclaimers

This book and the information herein is the result of intensive research over a decade. The information was gathered from an inordinate number of sources. The reader is advised not to take any information with anything but casual observation for educational purposes. Although some information was derived from scientific sources, readers must not assume that any of the content of this book or of any scientific sources are necessarily true or accurate. Errors are often found in peer-reviewed research publications. Science is evolving, and misinterpretations and misapplied data occurs in the scientific sector.

Readers are encouraged to research the topic of tickborne infections to keep abreast of the evolving science. Any references to any organizations or persons in this book are purely illustrative. Such references pertain *only* to the individual(s) from the named entity who are/were involved in the specific topic of discussion. No other inferences or connections are made or should be assumed. There are no allegations made or intended as to right or wrong actions by any persons, groups, institutions, or agencies; and none should be assumed.

In some areas of this book, the author has employed emphasis to statements in the form of underscored, bolded, or italicized type. Some published research was found in various texts that although it was not cited directly, it was sometimes used to help uncover additional resources. The author thanks any unnamed contributors.

The author is *not* a healthcare professional, scientist; nor someone with specific training in medicine. The author cannot, and is not providing any medical advice nor recommendations for the prevention, diagnosis, or treatment of any disease nor medical condition. Do not rely upon any information or ideas in this book as medical advice. Always seek the advice of a qualified medical practitioner before undertaking any therapy or change in therapy. This material is a collection of ideas based upon a study of a significant body of research. It is presented solely for informational purposes and independent study. There is no guarantee of accuracy made or implied in any portion of these materials in any of their formats.

Acknowledgments

To God, I am your humble servant and messenger. A special thank you to those who support me. A personal thank you to Lyme treating physicians and practitioners, for your dedication to a denied population in the face of adversity. Thank you to David Roth and the Tick-Borne Disease Alliance (TBDA), to Scott, Dawn Birling, Dolores Claesson, Catherine Back, Pam Thomson, Dr. Mike Maddox Dr. Joseph Jemsek, Marc Neuman, Christine Heidt, Jennie Burke, Lucia Cargill, Amanda Elam, Dr. Andrew Ladhams, Susan Green, and Nancy Mackay. To my children, my love always. Thank you to the individuals and publications who granted permission to reprint and to any other contributors not mentioned herein.

It is especially for those who do not believe in the persistence of tickborne infections, for those who do know but who fail to publicly acknowledge them, and for those who do not have any information at all that this booklet has been written.

Purpose

The purpose of this book is to help patients, physicians, legislators, and others recognize, test for, and/or approach treating tickborne illnesses. These include Lyme, Morgellons, Southern Tick-Associated Rash Illness, and a group of additional infections (co-infections). Co-infections are transmitted in addition to Lyme and the so-called "Morgellons," or sometimes alone. This booklet is written in simple terms for people without medical training. If you desire more information, please write to the author's address at the front of this book.

Since ticks are tiny, most patients have no idea they were bitten or that they may carry tickborne infections. When ill patients seek help from a physician without training in tickborne infections, they may be misdiagnosed. This is because most tickborne infections mimic other illnesses. Some doctors recognize a few Lyme symptoms, but most will be missed because tickborne infection testing and education is limited.

Lyme and other tickborne infections are often misdiganosed as Multiple Sclerosis (MS), Alzheimer's disease, Amyotrophic Lateral Sclerosis (ALS), Parkinson's, Lupus, Rheumatoid Arthritis, Fibromyalgia, Myalgic Encephalomyelitis (ME), Depression, or even delusional parasitosis.

Tickborne illness education is sorely needed. This booklet will help readers learn about tickborne infections around the world. While this information evolves over time, there is evidence to prove that untreated tickborne infections are serious, debilitating, and sometimes deadly.

Decades ago doctors repeatedly told me, "there is no Lyme disease in Wisconsin." This unfortunate stance was due to a lack of education about important global infections. Today there is no reason to be uninformed about tickborne diseases. Patients should no longer have to wait years to be correctly diagnosed and treated.

I was first infected with Lyme in 1969 in Illinois. My children and I were bitten in Wisconsin in 1992. I was rebitten in 2000. It was not until 2004 that we were all correctly diagnosed with Lyme and co-infections. By then I was partially paralyzed. I now have nerve damage, severe allergies, and persistent infections despite multiple antibiotics over decades. Had our infections been recognized earlier, our treatments would have been minimal and successful.

Our family, friends, and animals have tick-borne infections. In some states and countries, most neighbors are infected. Many people have been ill for so long, they have no idea how long it will take to become well. The longer one goes without treatment, the more expensive and lengthy it becomes. Specialized tick-borne disease tests are costly; and so are long-term treatments, lost wages, and other costs. People should not be fearful of tick-borne infections. They should be informed about prevention and take precautions to avoid becoming infected. If bitten, they should seek medical attention at the earliest sign of symptoms to be promptly and successfully treated.

Physicians who treat tick-borne infections face disinformation and discrimination as many public health experts lack current information about these infections. An era of silence blankets tick-borne diseases, which for decades has slowed the spread of information from within the halls of top research laboratories. It is time for this information to be revealed so patients can be aware of what they are facing, and so that physicians can be the true healers they are intended to be.

- PJ Langhoff

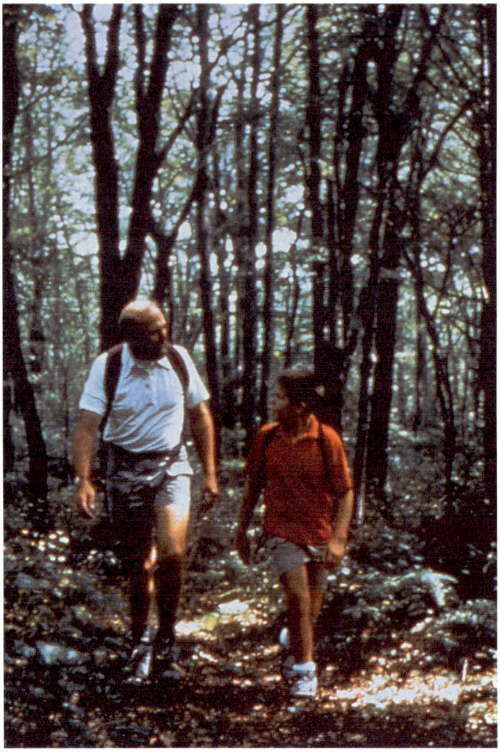

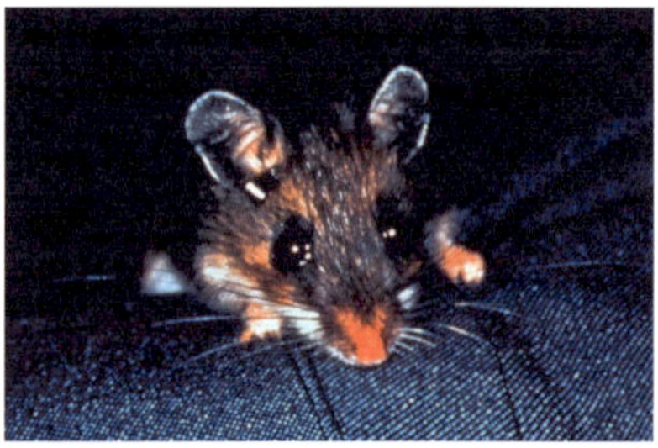

Above: *Peromyscus leucopus*, the white footed-mouse, a major host of Lyme disease and ticks. Migratory birds are also major hosts of ticks that carry Lyme disease. CDC Image.

Left: Woodlands and trails are prime tick habitats. It is important to wear protective clothing, tick repellants, and to stay in the middle of trails. Use caution when walking in tall grass, brush; or when in contact with tree limbs or woody plants. It is important to check yourself, family members, friends, and pets after being outdoors if you have visited, or live in an area that is likely to have ticks. CDC image.

Below: Deer are a main host of Lyme transmitting ticks, even in the winter. Ticks can remain active even in very cold temperatures. Some adult ticks can go years without a blood meal. Image PJ Langhoff.

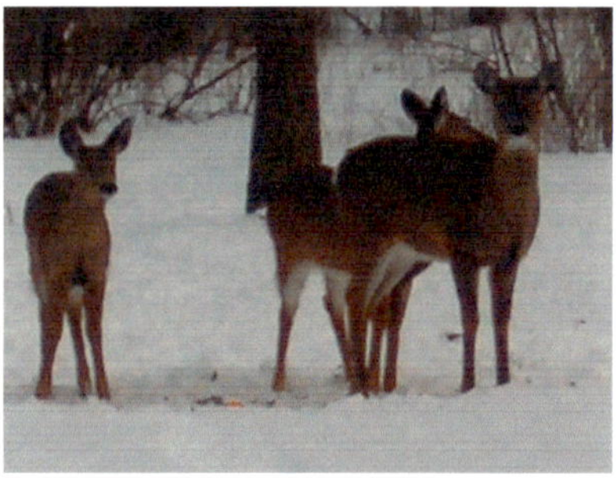

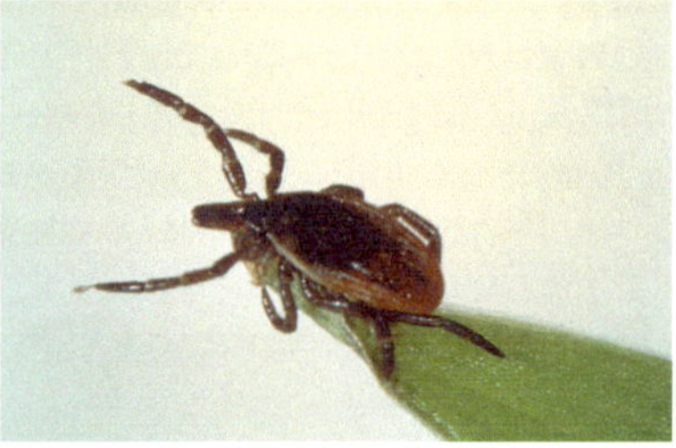

Above: An adult black-legged (*Ixodes scapularis*) tick "questing" upon a grass blade. Ticks waves their front legs about and grab hold of passing animals or humans for a blood meal. They will crawl to a warm, dark place; prefering the neck, scalp, behind the ear, armpit, groin, and behind the knee. Image CDC/Anna Perez.

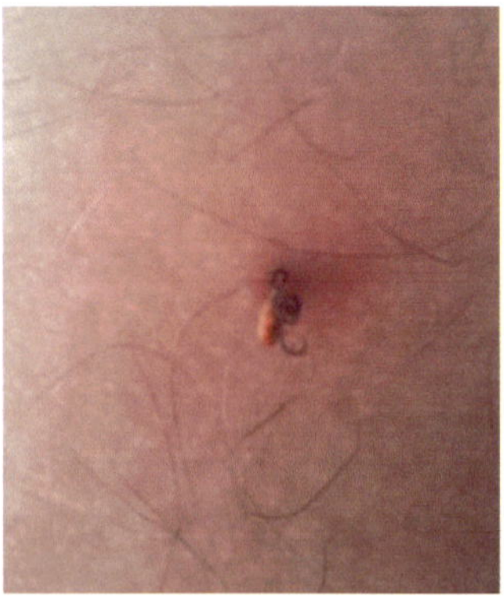

Right: An embedded black-legged *Ixodes scapularis* hard-bodied (deer) tick found on a Wisconsin patient. Note head down feeding position with mouth parts buried underneath the skin. It takes just minutes to attach. Image Dawn Birling.

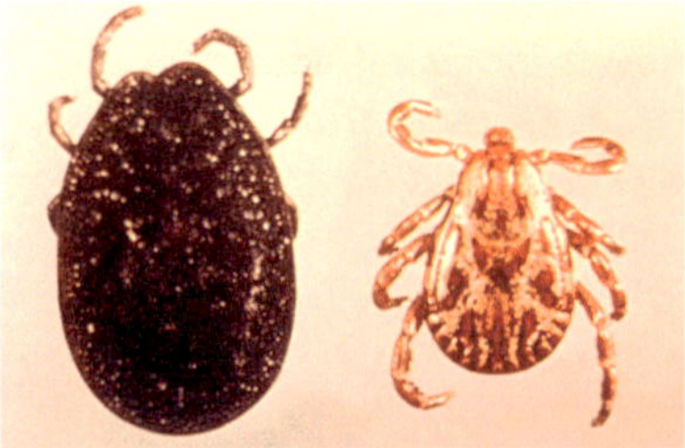

Far Left: Soft-bodied *Argasid* tick, near left: Hard-bodied *Ixodes* tick. CDC image.

One: Recognizing Tickborne Infections

What are Ticks and What is Lyme Disease?

Lyme disease is an infection that is transmitted by a tick, which is an *arthropod* ("arthro" means "jointed legs"). Infectious diseases are transmitted by many arthropods including ticks, mites, spiders, and lice; as well as by insects. *Tickborne illnesses* are infectious diseases that are transmitted by any of a species of *soft-bodied* or *hard-bodied* ticks.

Ticks live in all areas of the world. They are blood feeders which target reptiles, birds, animals, and humans. Common prey are livestock, field mice, raccoons, rabbits, squirrels, birds, and deer. They thrive in moist, warm areas such as forests, wood piles; and areas where ground cover includes wet leaves or tall grass. They do not thrive in dry areas.

Ticks have tiny mouth parts which act like scissors. Their bites are often painless since their saliva can have an antiseptic to conceal the bite. Ticks are delicate in weight and tiny. Unless an adult tick crawls upon bare flesh, it may be unseen or noticed only during feeding.

There are two families of ticks, the soft-bodied *Argasidae*, and the hard-bodied *Ixodidae*. Ticks feed in daylight or at night. Soft-bodied ticks latch on, take a quick blood meal, and drop off after feeding. Hard-bodied ticks attach for several days by "cementing" their head under the skin where they remain during the entire meal before dropping off.

Ticks have four life stages: egg, larval, nymph, and adult. After hatching they typically take a single blood meal in each stage before molting to the next. They find prey by crawling or by "questing" (holding onto grass or leaves). There they extend their front legs to latch onto passing prey. They also find prey by detecting expelled carbon dioxide (CO_2).

Despite some reports, **ticks are able to transmit human infections before, and immediately upon attachment, not 24-72 hours later.**[1,24,25,165] Tickborne infections are found within a tick's mid-gut; in its saliva, on and in its body, its excrement, and upon its contaminated hypostome (tool to pierce flesh). A female tick ovipositor (egg laying structure) also transmits infections to eggs as they are laid, so larval ticks are born infected. **Patients are sometimes *prophylactically* treated (preventively before symptoms) after a tick bite. Patients without evidence of a bite are usually treated only if symptoms appear.**

Previous page, bottom far right: Ticks use their mouth parts to break the skin. Some species inject an anesthetic into the skin to disguise the bite. They bury their head under the skin, and "cement" themselves with a fluid to feed over a period of days. A tick's body expands many times in size to engorgement. Once feeding ends, they detach and fall off the host.

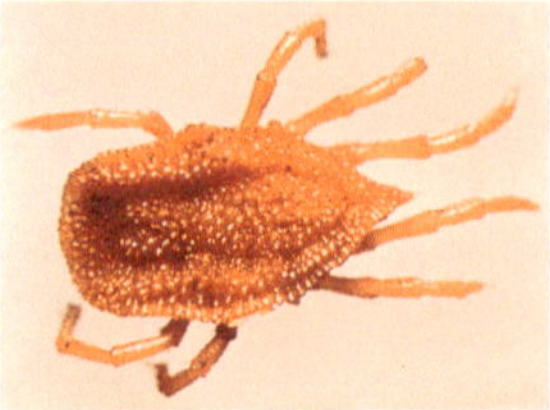

Before I had Lyme disease, I had never seen a tick!

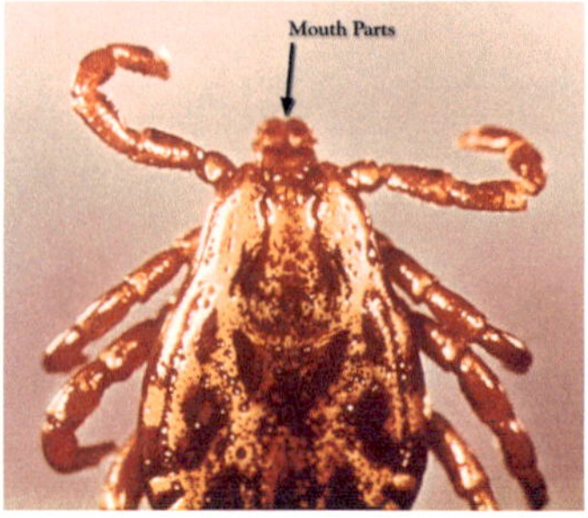

Above (L): Argasid (soft-bodied) tick. Right: Mouth parts of an *Ixodes* (hard-bodied) tick. Below: The microscopic spirochete of Lyme disease, *Borrelia burgdorferi.* CDC images.

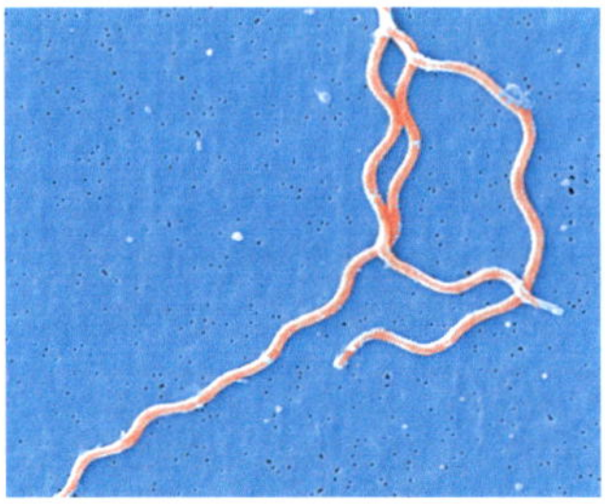

Right: Three black-legged *Ixodes scapularis* ticks. Left to right: nymph, adult, and larva. Larval ticks are only slightly larger than a poppy seed. CDC image.

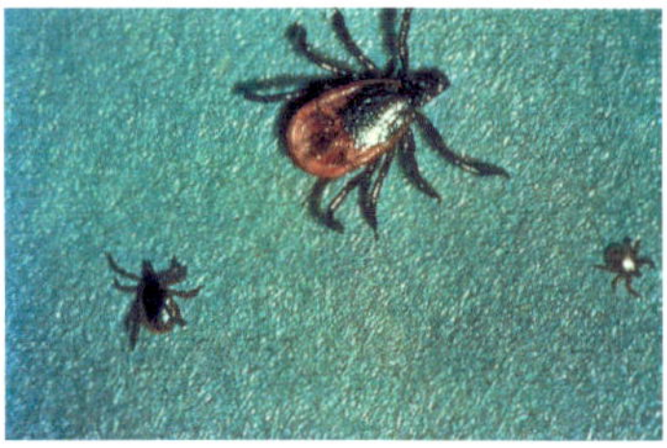

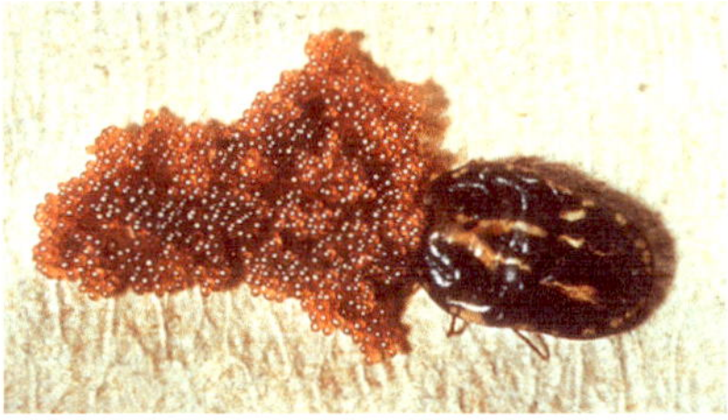

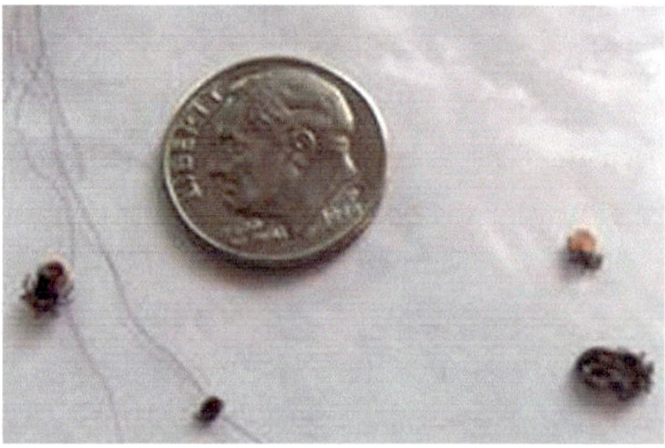

Above: Female *Ixodes* tick lays eggs and will soon die. Soft tick females lay many batches of eggs. CDC image. Right: *Ixodes* ticks in various sizes including nymph, adult, and engorged adult. There are over 200 species of *Ixodes* ticks. Many transmit Lyme disease to humans, as well as other co-infections. Image Dawn Birling.

The infectious agent of Lyme disease is called *Borrelia burgdorferi,* or "Bb." It is a *spirochete*; a spiral-shaped bacteria too small to see. "Borrelia" means tick-transmitted. The name "burgdorferi" refers to Dr. Willy Burgdorfer, the scientist credited with discovering the agent.

Lyme disease is also called *Lyme Borreliosis.* "Bb" is a curious organism. As a spirochete, it burrows through skin, cartilage, and other soft tissues; as well as bone and blood vessels. Bb spirochetes have also been detected in animal and human blood cells called *macrophages*.[2-4]

Bb is reported to be a "Gram-negative" organism for how it stains in the laboratory. It actually stains weakly Gram-positive. This may be a hint that tickborne infection treatments should address this difference.

Bb spirochetes assume several different forms including *motile* (moving), cyst, bleb, granule, gemma, spheroplast L, and other forms. Bb persists inside the body despite antibiotics. This has been demonstrated even in patients who test negative for Lyme disease (seronegative). Bb hides within slimy *biofilms* where it is protected from internal temperatures and chemical changes (i.e. fevers/herbs/antibiotics). Many bacteria use communal biofilms in the body and in the environment for protection.

Bb grows slowly, and only a single spirochete will produce disease. Bb assumes various forms and hides in the body to survive. It may be important to treat suspected Lyme patients *for as long as they have symptoms;* and not just for a limited 30-day or less period.[165]

Although Bb begins as a local skin infection, other infections that are transmitted by a tick bite can enter and infect us during tick feeding and upon contact. Therefore it may be highly valuable to treat patients using a *combination of antibiotics* which target *intracellular* (inside the cell) as well as *extracellular* (outside the cell) spaces. This offers a one-two punch to what are often multiple infections; and a treatment tactic which may provide patients with a more rapid and complete cure.

As with most illnesses, Lyme patients should be diagnosed *based upon clinical symptoms* and tick bite exposure risk. Many tickborne illness patients are misdiagnosed with Lupus, Crohn's, Rheumatoid Arthritis, Multiple Sclerosis, Fibromyalgia, Chronic Fatigue/ME, or other disorders.

Some physicians rely heavily upon CDC-recommended (standardized) laboratory tests to diagnose patients. This may not help many patients who have active tickborne infections. Standardized lab tests for Lyme disease are unreliable for most Bb strains, and cannot detect any coinfections at all. The CDC recommended two-tier tests include an ELISA (Enzyme-linked immunosorbent assay) and a Western blot (WB).

There are over 300 known Bb strains in the world. The three main Bb groups or families are (Group 1) *Borrelia burgdorferi* sensu lato (broad sense); (Group 2) *Borrelia garinii* (species novel); and (Group 3) *Borrelia afzelii.* Group 1 includes American and European strains. Group 2 includes strains from Europe and Asia, (a few strains have been detected in North America). Group 3 has European and Asian strains. A few North American patients have *B. afzelii* or *B. garinii* strains but they never traveled abroad. Birds are the most common carriers of Lyme-transmitting ticks.There are also tickborne borrelia strains that are related to relapsing fevers. These are "almost" Bb strains (*B. miyamotoi, B. lonestari, B. japonica, B. andesonii*), but they probably lack a key component found in typical Bb strains.[46,183]

The good news is that better Lyme testing is emerging. Newer diagnostic tests are far better at detecting existing tickborne infections over decades-old "standards." Newer tests can detect infections in seronegative Lyme patients, and there are many good specialty labs available. I have a list of some of these labs in the back of this book. Some public health and infectious disease personnel have claimed that some of these tests are "unproven" or "unvalidated." These claims are not necessarily true. Research and anecdotal evidence proves these tests aid in diagnosing tickborne infections. Many patients with ongoing symptoms even after previous antibiotics are found to be positive for Lyme and other tickborne infections using these newer tests. When retreated with antibiotics or other therapies, many of these patients are able to recover.

A Window of Opportunity

Tickborne infections are significantly on the rise around the world. Physicians must understand that the Centers for Disease Control (CDC) and other public health definitions for reporting Lyme disease cases are solely for public health use. Public health agencies try to estimate and track what are generally defined as "confirmed" human infection cases.

> *Patient infections should not be excluded from a diagnosis of Lyme disease if they do not meet public health surveillance case definitions!*

According to the CDC:

"Lyme disease is diagnosed based on symptoms, physical findings (e.g., rash), and the possibility of exposure to infected ticks."[47]

Patients who display a few, but not all symptoms described within CDC case definitions are often not reported as "confirmed" (valid) cases. Many Lyme cases are only reported months or years after initial infection. These cases are often diagnosed by physicians away from the area where the patient received a tick bite. Many infections are never reported, and many cases are misdiagnosed; including patients who test negative for Lyme but who are nevertheless Lyme infected.

The reasons for seronegativity are complex. The Bb organism can discard its outer "coat" to fool the immune system during acute infection. Some people make antibodies only weeks or months after becoming infected. Antibodies (when present), may be joined (complexed) with bacteria so none are free in a sample to be detected by a laboratory test. It can also take weeks to a month before spirochetes move from the skin (bite site) to the blood stream where they may be cultured from blood.

A blood test may produce a "false negative" result. This may occur if a patient is infected but no antibodies are detected by test probes. Only after some patients are treated with antibiotics are infection levels reduced to a point whereby antibodies may be detected by subsequent tests. Some culture tests require weeks before spirochetes can be detected, as Bb grows slowly. Interpreted too early, such tests will be "negative." It is unkind to make patients wait weeks to begin treatments that can eliminate infections long before test results arrive.

Some laboratory tests produce a "false positive" result. This is really a reflection of the test's limitations, or is caused by improper interpretation. Positive results usually mean that the patient is positive for the agent being tested. Sometimes however if a test is very limited in its ability to detect Bb, then a "false positive" may occur. Patients with an "equivocal" result simply do not meet a positive cut-off point. It does not mean that they are necessarily negative for Lyme disease. Again if a test is unclear whether it has detected Bb, then another test may be in order.

There is such a thing as a "false negative" result. Some patients are seronegative no matter what kind of test is used. It does not necessarily mean that they do not have Lyme disease or other tickborne infections. No single test can detect every strain of Lyme disease. Patients benefit from diagnostic tests which look for *multiple* Bb strains over those able to detect only one or two. A "negative" or "false positive" does not mean the patient is not infected, although it rarely could. It is important to always diagnose patients based on *symptoms and tick exposure*, and to use laboratory tests only to confirm, and not to diagnose patients.

For decades, public health officials have relied upon reported case numbers to educate the public about tickborne infections. When case numbers appear low, public education is not a high priority. However patients contract infectious diseases that do not follow carefully defined statistics. Patient infections go unreported, unrecognized, and most importantly, untreated or under treated. The huge disparity of opinion between *actual* case numbers and *reported* case numbers of tickborne infections is largely due to a lack of reliable information and reporting.

We must focus on how to *properly* identify tickborne infections. Many patients are told they only have a "spider bite." Patients historically wait an average of several years before they receive an accurate diagnosis of Lyme and/or other tickborne infections. This leaves patients to suffer much longer from illnesses that are more easily treated during the acute stage.

There is a narrow window of opportunity following a tick bite whereby tickborne infections can be easily and successfully treated using a minimum of medicines. This period falls within the first few days to a week following a tick bite (not a month). Some public health officials suggest that patients should be "observed" for a period of a month after a tick bite to see if they produce symptoms before any treatment begins. This approach has proven devastating for most patients since tick populations are heavily infected with numerous agents. Unchecked human infections quickly spread throughout the body where they thereafter hide in places that antibiotics cannot easily penetrate.[25]

The best chance tickborne infection patients have of successful treatment is *within the first few days following a tick bite.* The longer a patient must wait for a proper diagnosis and treatment, the more entrenched these infections become. Delayed diagnosis and treatment allows more damage to occur in the body. Such delays necessitate extended treatment durations and their associated increased costs.

Lyme Disease is a Complex, Serious Infection

It is clear from many sources that Lyme disease is, and for many years has been understood to be a *serious, potentially chronic infection that does not always respond to antibiotic treatments.* It is curious then why the words "Lyme disease" have become so political. Important statements may be learned from a 2002 patent invention:[5]

> *"The infection, if untreated, commonly persists for months to years despite the occurrence of host antibody and cellular responses; this observation indicates effective evasion of the immune response. Lyme disease may be disabling (particularly in its chronic form.)"*

This is vital information that physicians need to know. Here is another patent with equally important revelations:[6]

> *"Lyme disease may be missed or misdiagnosed when it does appear...At present, all stages of Lyme disease are treated with antibiotics. Treatment of early disease is usually effective, however the cardiac, arthritic, and nervous system disorders associated with the later stages often do not respond to therapy."*

This last quote came from the text of a 1994 patent. Its authors mentioned a 1989 study of Rheumatologist Dr. Allen C. Steere, one of the first physicians to investigate a 1970's cluster of Connecticut Lyme patients. There are numerous older sources which tell us that Lyme disease has long been seen as a persistent, debilitating infection. This evidence proves that if Lyme disease is not treated *at onset*, it will progress to a chronic state that requires months or years to eliminate.[13,16,26-28]

Despite such knowledge at the highest levels of public health, physicians often misdiagnose patients who have tickborne infections. Consequently, untreated or under treated patients are also routinely denied disability and/or insurance coverage, especially for Lyme disease. This is often due to the over reliance upon published infectious disease guidelines for the diagnosis and treatment of tickborne infections. The most commonly cited guidelines are very limited in scope; addressing only a few tickborne infections in an acute form. They do not appear to properly address misdiagnosed or under treated tickborne infections.[29,30]

Doctors in many countries rely upon Lyme disease guidelines to help diagnose and treat patients. These guidelines recommend brief antibiotic therapy except for a subset of patients with ongoing symptoms. Well-meaning physicians mistakenly treat patients once for tickborne illnesses according to such guideline recommendations. Afterward they decline additional antibiotics and cite guideline recommendations, instead of relying upon a patient's progression and response to treatment. Infections do not know how to follow a calendar. There is no excuse to deny any treatment therapies to patients who suffer with ongoing symptoms.[29,30]

Patients have a reasonable right, and should ask physicians to offer treatments for longer periods to address continual symptoms for persistent infections. Unfortunately many physicians prefer to take a "safe" approach and will prescribe only a 30-day regimen; and only for new infections. This is a serious disservice to patients. It is also why some patients in declining health must turn to physicians who specialize in treating *chronic* tickborne infections. These physicians are often referred to as "Lyme literate" medical doctors. This means simply that they have more practical experience treating these highly complex illnesses.

"LLMDs" believe that tickborne infections are serious and debilitating for patients. A group of these highly skilled professionals belong to a medical society that promotes similar viewpoints. The society advocates a broader set of diagnostic and treatment guidelines for physicians to follow when handling patients who have tickborne illnesses.

These guidelines are available to download (at no cost) at the web site of the International Lyme and Associated Diseases Society (www.ILADS.org). It is the experience of physicians who follow these and similar practices, that when antibiotics are provided to patients in the right combination and for longer durations; the infections resolve or significantly improve for many patients. These guidelines also recognize that additional supportive therapies and specialized testing may be required to diagnose and treat patients who harbor complex tickborne infections.[10,31]

Insurers, disability agencies, and medical boards should consider that there is more than a single school of thought or set of guidelines to treat tickborne infections. Patients who are unable to work, and/or who require additional medical care deserve their benefits. Patients with tickborne infections are not "cases" to be "managed." They cannot be clearly defined using cost-saving corporate or government guidelines. Chronic, legitimate infections require special consideration. Patients need and deserve opportunities for extended care and financial support while disabled.

It makes little sense today for anyone not to admit that Lyme and other tickborne infections are often serious and persistent. This is especially true for patients who do not receive a timely diagnosis and adequate treatments. Sadly, some patients are accused of being "delusional" for believing they may remain infected after antibiotic therapy. These patients recognize their ongoing symptoms as disease. However a few physicians believe such symptoms to be nothing more than an "autoimmune" reaction to a previous infection. Persistent tickborne infections are what some have labeled to be a "post-Lyme syndrome."

Lyme disease was named after a Connecticut town where a cluster of patients were found (Old Lyme). Experts have known for decades that Lyme is a serious infection that may not respond to antibiotics. A Connecticut Rheumatologist was the first to suggest that patients *may* have an autoimmune disorder rather than ongoing infection. The theory at best appears only partly correct; but people continue to promote "post-Lyme syndrome."[32]

Patients with persisting symptoms have been tested years after multiple antibiotics. My blood for example, reveals *culturable Bb spirochetes.* I am negative by CDC standardized tests for Lyme. It cannot be argued that I have nothing but an autoimmune reaction years later without subsequent exposure, when living spirochetes are detectable in my blood.

Long-term antibiotics are helpful if you ask Lyme patients and their physicians. A recent, limited study concluded that long-term antibiotics have little to no benefit for Lyme patients. However the reality is that Lyme patients achieve wellness using longer or repeated treatment programs. Some of these therapies include the administration of pulsed and combined antibiotics; as well as other supportive nutritional, detoxification, oxygenation, antibody, methylation, and/or endocrine therapies.[7]

Signs of Acute Lyme Disease Infection

The next page shows some examples of the kinds of rashes that may appear in some Lyme patients. Not all patients develop a rash, and not all rashes have the distinctive (hallmark) "bull's-eye" appearance.

Various Lyme rashes. Size and appearance varies and may be hard for physicians to recognize. Rashes are generally not painful. Patients may have none, singular, multiple, or repetitive rashes.

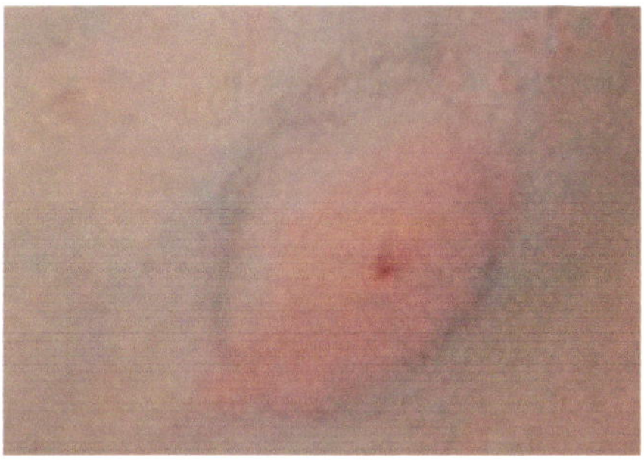

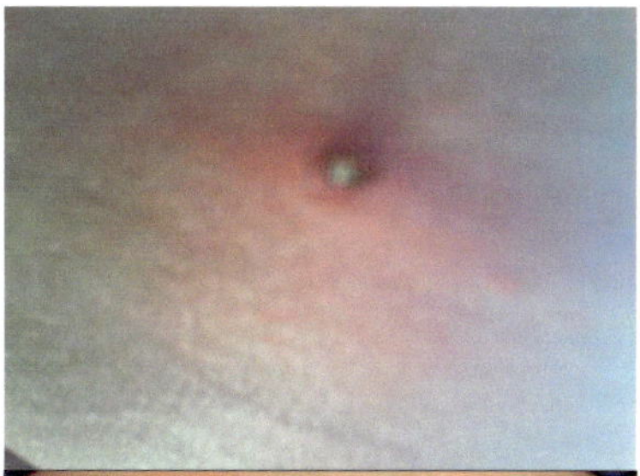

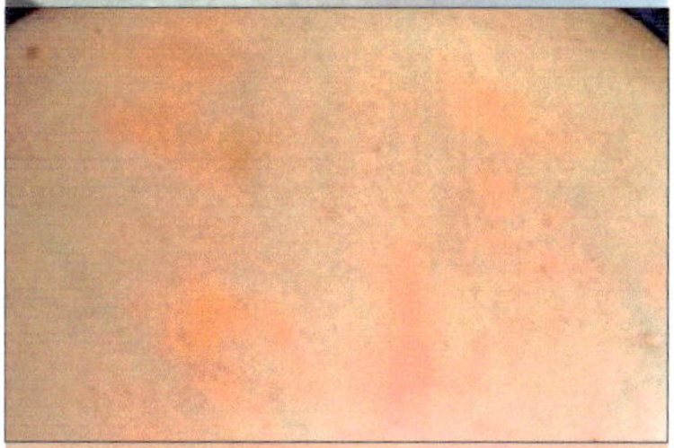

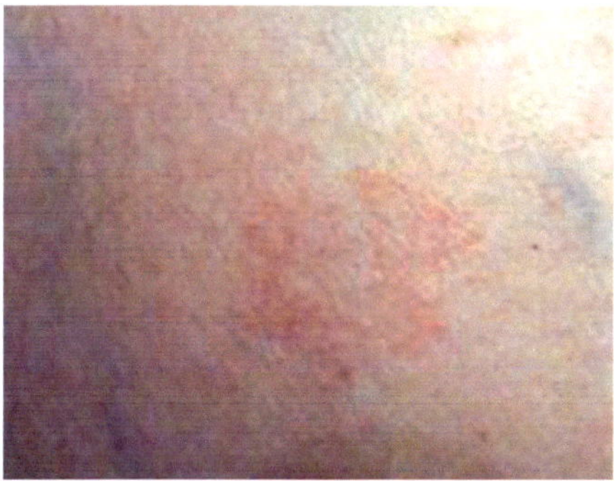

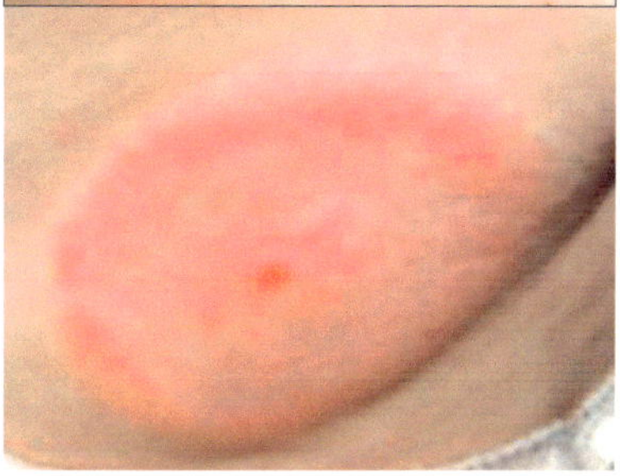

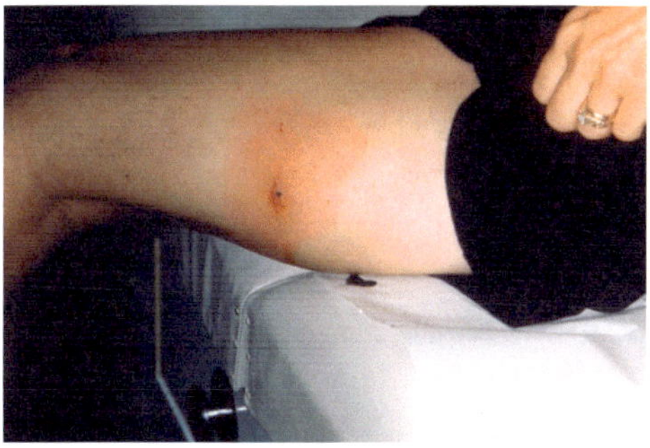

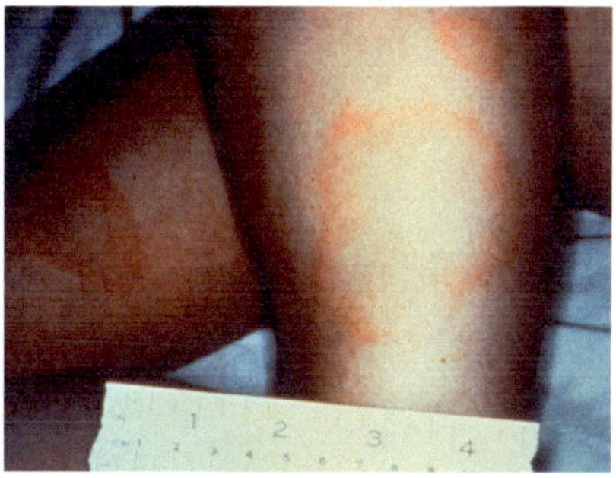

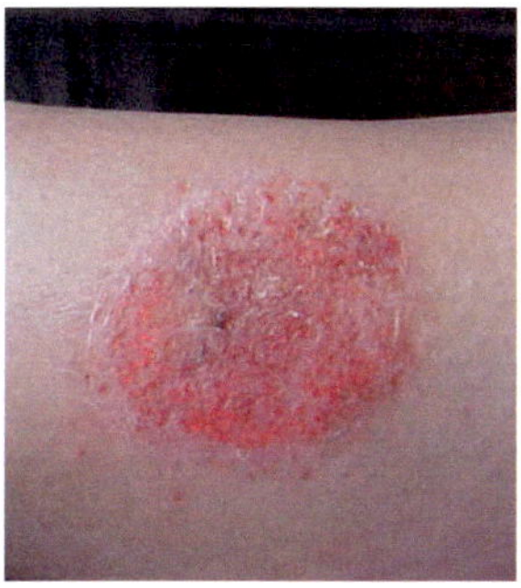

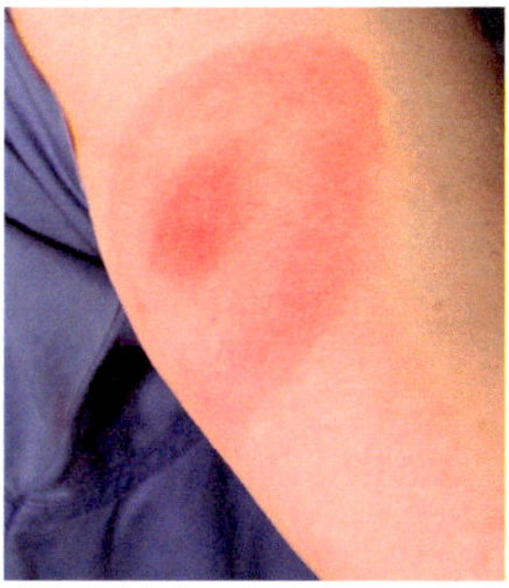

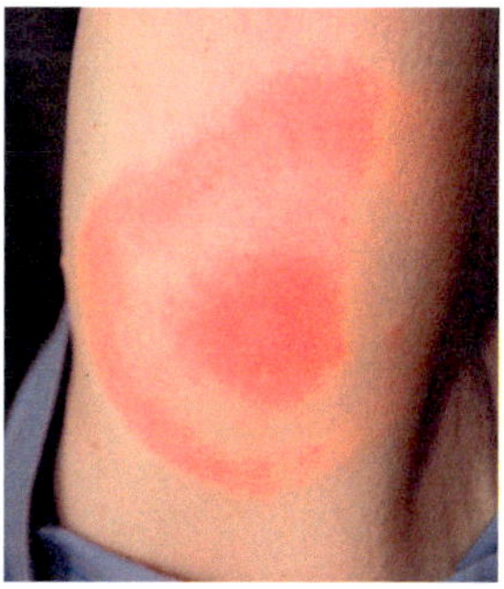

All images this page: Dawn Birling except bottom middle and bottom right are CDC/Anna Perez.

During acute Lyme infection, along with other physical symptoms, approximately 30-40% of patients have some kind of rash. Typical cases have a central bite mark where the tick fed or was removed. (Be sure to remove any remaining mouth parts if seen.) A small area of redness forms around the bite mark. This is called an *Erythema migrans* (EM) rash. "Erythema" means "red" and "migrans" means to migrate or to go away. It is also called an *Erythema chronicum migrans* (ECM) rash.

The rash expands outwardly over days. There may be a flesh colored area inside a red circle, lending a "bull's-eye" (target) appearance. A bull's-eye rash is a hallmark symptom of acute Lyme infection. Rashes disappear without treatment, but this does not "cure" the patient.

The disappearance of a rash reveals that the infection has spread beyond the skin into other parts of the body. Some people never have a rash. Others have plain, blotchy, or multiple smaller rashes which appear elsewhere; and occasionally reappear. Days or weeks later, additional rashes may emerge alone or in multiples anywhere on the body. They may present as rings or blotches that are round, oval, or simple and vague red areas. Patients can have Lyme and other tickborne infections without ever having any kind of a rash. Person-to-person transmissions occur, especially mother-to-child (in utero) transmission. Tickborne infections can be transmitted through contaminated human body fluids (i.e. saliva, breast milk, blood, and urine).[165]

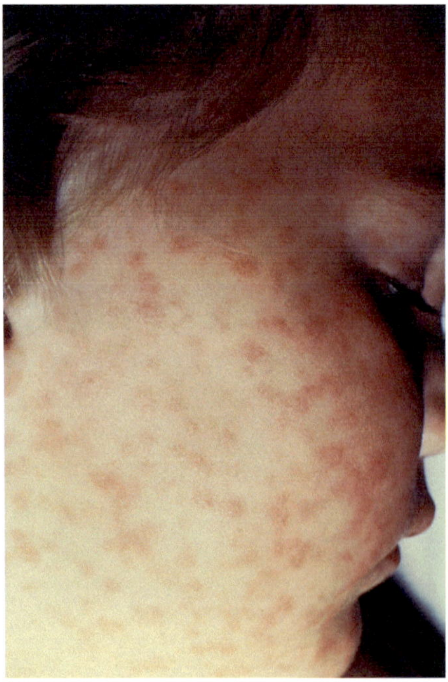

Other types of rashes may appear. These may be caused by other serious infections such as Rocky Mountain spotted fever. This rash has a distinct spotted appearance. Suspected cases should seek immediate medical attention.

Tick exposures should be discussed with a physician. Be sure to recall recent travel, occupation, recreation, pets, and home habitat. Physicians should not rely upon maps or case numbers to decide infection risk. Patients are often bitten in areas not felt to be endemic (highly prevalent) for tickborne diseases.

Left: A child with the characteristic rash of *Rocky Mountain spotted fever,* a serious tickborne infection that can be fatal. CDC image.

Common Tickborne Illness Symptoms

Ticks are very small. Unless a patient removes an engorged tick from their body, they may be completely unaware they have been bitten. During the first stage of acute infection, most patients who have been bitten by an infected tick manifest flu-like symptoms. If a "flu" occurs during the summer, Lyme disease should be suspected even if no bite is recalled. Tickborne infections typically begin with moderate and migrating pains, malaise, and fatigue. Depending upon the infections carried by the tick, symptoms may remain mild, or rapidly progress to serious illness.

The most commonly reported symptoms of many acute tickborne infections are similar. Infections may include the following symptoms. These may be produced by Lyme alone, or by any combination of additional infections (co-infections). It is important for patients to tell physicians if they suspect or are aware they have had a tick bite.

- Characteristic circular "bull's-eye" rash at bite site which spreads outward
- Rashes in other parts of the body, not necessarily ring-shaped
- Any size or shape rash that is not necessarily itchy or painful
- Sore throat and/or flu-like symptoms, especially in the summer
- Mild or severe headaches or migraines; unexplained head or sinus pressure
- Unexplained hair loss, scalp or skin becomes painful to the touch
- Twitching of facial muscles or other muscles; facial paralysis or Bell's palsy
- Tingling or numbness of facial muscles, or any part of the body
- Unexplained pain in jaw or neck, swollen glands
- Pain or swelling in or around the eyes
- Vision changes; light sensitivity, uveitis, conjunctivitis, increased "floaters"
- Reduced hearing; ear pain; ringing or buzzing sounds; tinnitis
- Hypersensitivity to sound or easily overwhelmed by sound or movement
- Joint pain or swelling; pain migrates throughout the body
- Muscle cramps, stiffness in muscles or joints
- Irritable digestion, diarrhea, nausea, vomiting, constipation, gut dysbiosis
- Painful chest, back, ribs, or other bones
- Shortness of breath or "air hunger"
- Heart block, arrythmia; palpitations, extra or missed beats
- New panic attacks or unexplained anxiety, paranoia
- Night sweats; unexplained fevers (high or low) or chills
- Shaking, tremors, feeling of vibration or being jittery
- Burning, stabbing, or insect bite-like pains in the body
- Weakness, fainting; balance or coordination problems
- Partial or complete paralysis on one or both sides of the body
- Loss of speech or motor skills; trouble speaking and/or swallowing
- Dizziness, vertigo; difficulty walking

- Postural hyper- or hypotension/rapid blood pressure changes on position change
- Tingling sensations or pinpricks, especially in extremities
- Lightheadedness, woozy feeling or increased motion sickness
- Hypersensitivity to movement; loss of awareness of body in time or space
- Mood swings, irritability, sudden outbursts, rage; new compulsive behaviors
- Unusual or sudden depression, irritability, suicidal/homicidal thoughts
- New frequent nightmares (adults), night terrors (children), sleepwalking
- Incontinence; loss of bladder function/control; nightly trips to bathroom
- Visual or auditory hallucinations (seeing/hearing imaginary things/sounds)
- Disorientation and memory problems; feeling or easily getting lost
- Feeling of "losing your mind"; scattered thinking, loss of concentration
- Confusion; communication issues, trouble following conversations, dementia
- Slurred/slowed speech; stammering; dyslexic speech or writing
- Going to the wrong place; forgetting how to perform simple tasks
- Loss of interest in sex; sexual dysfunction
- (Females) Unexplained menstrual issues, pelvic pain, breast pain/discharge
- (Males) Testicular or pelvic pain
- Unexplained weight gain or loss; sudden change in appetite
- Sudden allergies to foods, chemicals, and other substances
- Extreme fatigue; daytime or excessive sleepiness or insomnia
- Nystagmus, arthritis, hydrocephaly, especially in children
- Change in overall body temperature (too high/too low)
- A flu that you had but after which you never seem to recover[35-41]

As we can see, many of these symptoms are found in an assortment of medical conditions. It is no wonder that physicians may have a difficult time detecting acute tickborne infections in patients. This is especially true if the patient does not recall a tick bite or if there was no rash seen.

Lyme disease is called "the new great imitator." Its symptoms mimic many other illnesses. With a tick bite, any number of infectious agents may be transmitted. Ticks are "dirty" creatures since they feed upon wild and domestic animals before spreading infections to humans.

Physicians, please entertain the possibility that infectious diseases may be a part of your patient's illness. Insect-borne infections are commonplace throughout the world, although they are seldom considered as a source of acute symptoms in patients.

If a patient claims not to feel well despite antibiotics or other treatments, then please assume that the patient is telling the truth. Most people have better things to do than to visit numerous doctors simply to complain about the "aches and pains" of daily living. In a truly healthy patient, no aches or pains should ever be found.

Symptoms of Disseminated Infection

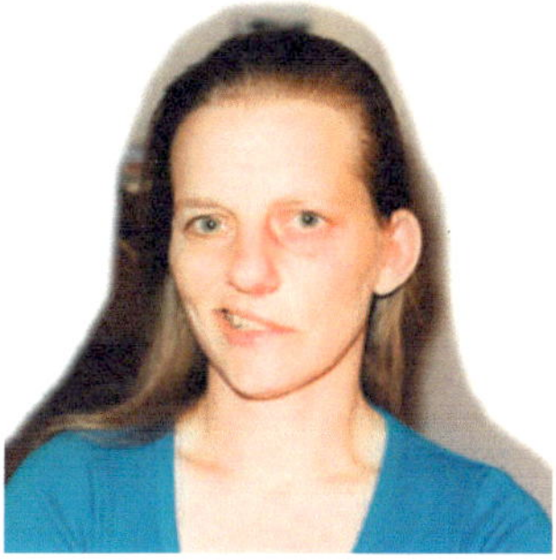

Left: The author in 2000 with left sided Bell's palsy and *Borrelial Lymphocytoma* of left ear (swelling, redness). Note droopy eyelid. Duration of palsy was 9 weeks. Treatment was intramuscular Rocephin. The patient had temporary loss of multiple cranial nerves (forehead, left, middle areas of the face, no sense of smell or taste). There was difficulty eating and swallowing. Pain from scalp to left ear, jaw, neck, shoulder and mid-back.

Multiple misdiagnoses included shingles of the cranial nerve without pustules, spider bite, virus, and idopathic palsy. Five physicians in a Lyme-endemic state ignored the patient's indication that she had a tick bite. Bell's palsy is a common sign of early disseminated Lyme.

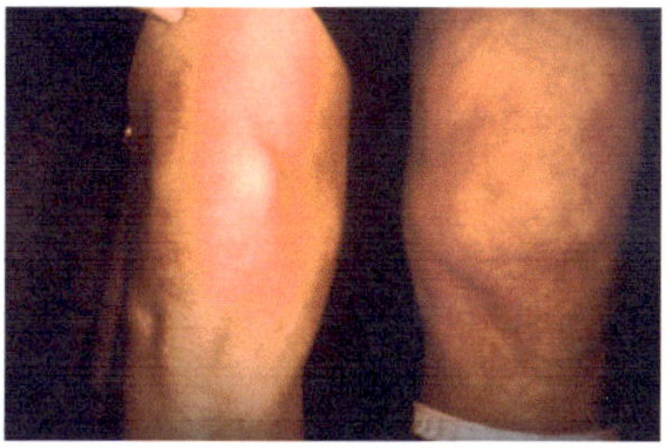

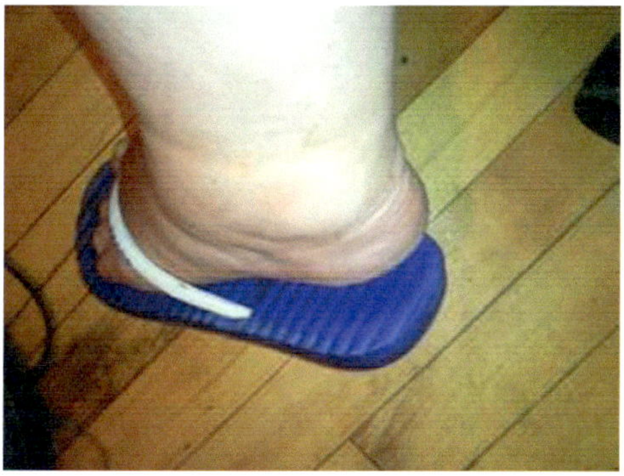

Above left: Swelling of a man's left knee from Lyme arthritis. Right: Swollen leg and ankle in a non-obese Lyme patient. Swelling may be severe or barely noticeable. Image CDC/Anna Perez.

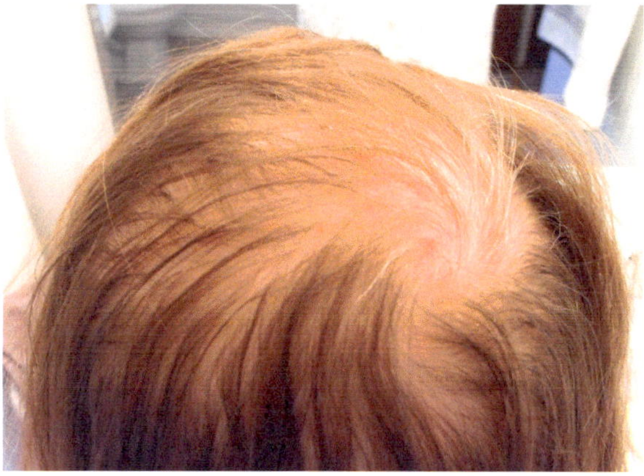

Left: 50 year old female Lyme patient with diffuse hair loss. Patient tested positive for antibodies to *Bartonella henselae, Borrelia burgdorferi,* and *Mycoplasma pneumoniae.*

Although the patient was not tested for antibodies to *Chlamydia pneumonia,* the hair loss pattern is consistent with other patients who test positive for the infection.

Low thyroid and "female" hormones also contribute to hair loss. Some patients with hair loss have supplemented their diet with biotin. Bb spirochetes are said to bind to collagen and to biotin in the body.[49,50]

What Do Chronic Tickborne Infections Look Like?

Once the Bb organism disseminates from the skin to the body, (a few days to a week), infection progresses to the second stage. Symptoms may continue from the initial infection; or cease only to surface *months to years* later. Rarely the second stage will appear a decade later. Generally speaking, symptoms grow steadily worse over time.

The second stage occurs either because the infection was untreated, or because some of the infection was resistant to treatment. Despite a myriad of symptoms, routine laboratory tests can return "normal" without obvious evidence of infections. Only special tickborne illness labs look for special markers to detect tickborne infections. The symptoms of "early" disseminated or second-stage Lyme disease are listed here, including those which continue from the acute or first stage.

- Bell's palsy (facial paralysis and drooping)
- Arthritic pain and loss of mobility, with or without joint swelling
- Neurological symptoms
- Buzzing sounds, tinnitis/ringing of the ears, hearing loss
- Poor balance and coordination, difficulty walking
- Irritability, depression, suicidal thoughts
- Paranoia, delusions, chronic depression, hypervigilance, OCD
- Hypersensitivities / new or increased allergies
- Meningitis, cranial neuritis or encephalitis
- Lesions in the white matter of the brain or organs (seen on SPECT or MRI)
- Seizures or strokes
- Marked and rapid hair loss (especially diffuse) in either sex
- Unexplained swollen glands, sore throat, chronic dry cough
- Paralysis or numbness, tingling or numbness in extremities
- Chronic gastritis, reflux, abdominal cramps, gut dysbiosis
- Irritable bladder or bowel, cystitis
- Visual and auditory disturbances, hallucinations
- Cognitive difficulties, confusion, dementia, memory problems
- Disorientation, going to the wrong place
- Rapidly changing eyesight, sudden reading difficulties
- Pain, swelling, or pressure behind eyes and sinuses
- Twitching or locking of facial or other muscles of the body
- Chest pains, difficulty breathing, shortness of breath
- Cardiovascular problems, arrhythmias, heart block
- Problems with speech, difficulty swallowing, gagging
- Sudden incontinence when there was no previous problem
- Menstrual problems, pelvic pain, testicular pain
- Sexual dysfunction, sudden loss of libido
- Obsessive compulsive behaviors, attention deficit disorders
- Personality disorders, bi-polar or irrational behavior, unusual argumentativeness
- Emotional lability

The numerous symptoms of early disseminated Lyme disease may confuse the most astute physicians. Once the initial symptoms (and rashes if any) disappear, Bb has entered into the central nervous system and/or other organ systems in the body besides the skin. This occurs hours, days, or weeks after initial infection. Symptoms may disappear for a time, or they may continue as the patient's health declines.

Chronic arthritis is commonly reported in patients with persistent infections. Neurologic problems occur in roughly half of infected patients.

Cardiac manifestations can appear chronically or only transiently along with neurologic, arthritic, or ocular (eye) symptoms; or any one symptom may be the only one noticed. Symptoms vary widely between patients, and are significantly impacted by stressors including surgery, injury, nutrition, immune function, emotional conflict, toxic metal burden, and the number and type of other infections present in the patient's body.

Some physicians prefer to perform a lumbar puncture (spinal tap) to rule out Lyme disease. This is a procedure that can sometimes indicate Lyme disease in a subset of patients. It should be carefully considered since the procedure is painful and risky; and Lyme or co-infections such as *Bartonella* may not always be evident in spinal fluid samples (CSF).

Spinal taps are not routinely recommended, and a negative tap does not rule out Lyme. Even in patients with meningitis, antibodies are found in the CSF in fewer than 13-20% of patients with acute or persistent Lyme. When taps are performed, some physicians look for elevated proteins and white cells, as well as other evidence of infective proteins.[8-10]

Another marker that is said to be useful is CXCL13. This is a marker for a protein that influences immune B cells. It is produced by the gut, liver, spleen, and lymph nodes during infection. This is a key marker found in the "rare" autoimmune disease *Myasthenia gravis* (MG). Since MG is a neuromuscular disorder, the presence of this marker hints that MG may have a tickborne infection at its core.[55,56]

If Lyme infections remain untreated during stage two, then the third or *tertiary* stage of infection occurs. This is sometimes referred to as late stage, disseminated, or *chronic Lyme disease*. Some physicians do not believe that this form of Lyme disease even exists. By this stage (up to a month to a decade later), patients are seriously ill with obvious and debilitating symptoms which can be life-threatening and completely disabling. Some of the more obvious and serious symptoms include:

- Encephalomyelitis, encephalopathy, aseptic meningitis
- Painful radiculopathies, peripheral nerve palsies
- Chronic arthritis in one or more joints, particularly large joints
- Allergies, chemical sensitivities, nutritional deficiencies, metabolic syndromes
- Starvation, wasting, or Crohn's disease-like digestive issues
- Dysautonomia, Postural Orthostatic Tachycardia Syndrome (POTS)
- Vasculitis, thrombosis (blood clots, hypercoagulation)
- Tourette's-like syndrome, seizures
- Cancer (tickborne infections predispose patients to certain cancers)

Disseminated Lyme disease may occasionally contribute to psychiatric disorders (particularly depression and rage) since the organisms severely impact endocrine and hormone function. Disordered hormones and neurotransmitters may contribute to depression, bipolar states, panic attacks, schizophrenia, dementia, paranoia, anorexia nervosa, attention deficit disorders, autism, obsessive-compulsive disorders, hypervigilance, fearfulness, rage and sleep disorders, and/or a flat affect. The hypothalamus (base of brain) is a common target of tickborne infections.[35]

Patients with possible psychiatric disorders may benefit from a thorough screening for tickborne illnesses. If infected, symptoms may lessen or resolve after treatment. Antibiotics that penetrate the blood-brain barrier are most effective in patients with neurologic or neuropsychiatric issues. Some Lyme patients are diagnosed as depressed. Quite frequently, some physicians do not believe patients remain ill after treatment. Patients may be misdiagnosed with a delusional or conversion disorder; or as if they are depressed when they merely have persistent infections. Even so, some patients do benefit from very low-dose antidepressants which act upon dysfunctional neurotransmitters. This can temporarily improve mood, muscle pain, and certain neurologic symptoms in some patients.[13,16]

Tickborne agents produce toxic proteins called neurotoxins. Neurotransmitters (signaling nerves) and their associated chemicals (i.e. dopamine, serotonin, acetylcholine) are in disarray during chronic infections. Misfiring nerves can alter sleep patterns, brain and muscle function; and cause chronic overstimulation and central and autonomic nervous system irritability. This can upset blood pressure, breathing, balance, body temperature, digestion, and other body clock functions (circadian rhythm).

In tickborne infections, physicians sometimes treat to support proper neurotransmitter function. Ill patients may benefit from a rebalanced brain and body chemistry including amino acids and micronutrients to help the body heal. It is extremely important to eliminate toxins that are produced by infectious agents; particularly during antibiotic treatments when die-off reactions may produce a temporary increase in symptoms.

In response to the presence of dying microbes, patients may experience a *Jarisch-Herxheimer* reaction (herx), and a resultant chemical (cytokine) storm. This temporary state significantly impacts symptoms, especially in patients with chronic infections. Unpleasant reactions are mediated with antihistamines, non-steroidal anti-inflammatories (NSAIDS), steam baths/saunas, lemon juice and olive oil drinks, enemas, or colonics to reduce ammonia levels; as well as other therapies. Severe "herxes" can be life-threatening, but most reactions are uncomplicated and short-lived.

Herxes are not immediate reactions. Rather they may emerge within hours or days of initial treatment. The duration varies from hours to days. Flares may erupt in tandem with the organism's growth cycle (roughly every four weeks), and symptoms may worsen during a flare. The intensity of herxes tends to decline as infection levels decline. Since antibiotics kill Bb during its growth phase, therapies may need to extend beyond a single calendar month to target newly growing organisms.

About one third of the population has a gene mutation which interferes with the important enzyme *Methylenetetrahydrofolate reductase* (MTHFR). This enzyme contributes to proper gene *methylation*, folic acid use, and breakdown of the amino acid *homocysteine*. It is responsible for the housekeeping of damaged genes and bacterial debris; and maintaining vitamin B, methionine, and SAMe levels. Genes are regulated by enzymes (methylation). Lyme patients are usually depleted of B, D, and other vitamins. Many benefit from liquid, sublingual, oral, or compounded vitamin injections.

Physicians might consider testing chronic Lyme patients for the MTHFR gene mutation. If present, it may have been damaged congenitally, by chemicals, by radiation, or by infections including tickborne illnesses. Deficiencies or elevations in this enzyme may lead to heart attacks, strokes, vein thrombosis (clots), inflammatory bowel disease, chronic disease, cancers, and neuropsychiatric symptoms.[11]

Proper detoxification of the body rapidly improves many physical and psychiatric symptoms, especially in people with tickborne infections and heavy metal, metalloid, or other toxic burdens. Patients may benefit from testing and removal of heavy metals and metalloids. Some clinics provide intravenous or oral detoxification protocols. In general, blood and challenge tests are better predictors than hair sampling. Most people carry a lifetime of multiple toxins in their bodies. People with chronic infections cannot remove these additional burdens. Excess toxins contribute to neurotoxicity.[12]

Tickborne infection symptoms also seem to improve when *fluorides* are removed from diet and healthcare products. *Fluorides and other chemicals can mutate bacteria including spirochetes*. Proper immune system and brain function begins within the gut. An overgrowth of toxic bacteria in the human gut must also be addressed. Important nutrients are carried throughout the body, so we literally are what we eat. When nutrients are depleted, enzymes cannot be produced, genes cannot express, damage cannot be repaired, and energy cannot be manufactured. Balancing gut function, detoxification, correcting diet, replenishing altered intestinal flora, and repairing nutrient and enzyme deficiencies are other important components of healing tickborne illnesses.[13,16]

Two: The Deeper Issues

Co-Infections: What Else Comes Along For the Ride?

Ticks are exposed to a number of environmental toxins. Chemical and *microbial insecticides* and industrial pollutants are of course the most common. Ticks crawl upon plants where they are exposed to natural and artificial spores, toxins, molds, viruses, and fungi. What they acquire there and during a blood meal from infected insects (i.e. moth larvae), or animals, birds, or reptiles determines which infections they transmit. The interactions between environmental microbes and what lies within a tick gut together contributes to human tickborne infections.[13,16]

Ticks exposures to microbial insecticides may play a pivotal role in tickborne infections. Insecticides are fed to, or applied to livestock animals, crops, and to forested areas. More recently, insecticides are being genetically engineered directly into plants to bypass the need for external pesticide applications. Insecticides are used in many industries.

During the 1850's, scientists began using insects, fungi, bacteria, and parasitizing insects to control insect pests upon agricultural crops, food stores, and livestock. Over time these techniques evolved to include chemicals. Once chemical pesticides fell by the wayside by 1970 due to their toxicity to wildlife and humans, the only insecticides which remained for use were largely those of a microbial nature.

These insecticides have also evolved over the past century and a half. I go into great depth about these in my tickborne infection books. It is not enough to simply know what such formulas contain. We need to understand how they impact targeted insect and arthropod populations; as well as their level of safety upon and within foods, animals, and humans.

The public may be interested to learn that an important soil bacteria has long been used as a microbial insecticide. This bacterium is closely related to the infectious agent called *Anthrax.* The bacteria, which is called *Bacillus thuringiensis* or "B.t." is used as a microbial insecticide. In the insect or arthropod body, it destroy gut cells and creates holes in the tissues. Latent infections would normally stay within gut cells and incapacitate or kill the insect or tick over a long period. Microbial insecticides which degrade gut tissues and deliver toxic lab-designed infections *significantly speed up the killing action of latent infections by reactivating and augmenting them.*

Ticks have a unique digestive process. They do not have stomach acids to kill natural or insecticidal microbes taken in during a meal. They directly digest their meals within their gut (epithelial) cells. From the mid-gut, ingested microbes make their way into the tick body. Once systemically infected, *a tick can expose a host to infections when feeding, regurgitating, or excreting wastes before, during, or after its blood meal.* A tick can infect a host simply *on contact,* and not just hours after a meal.[13,16,165-168]

The reactivation of latent infections in insects and arthropods is a desired goal of *genetically modified* (GM) microbial insecticides. Their specific purpose is to damage gut tissues, release GM toxins and microbes; and reactivate latent (intracellular) infections. They are highly toxic and efficient pest killers. Ticks that are systemically infected can and do spread infections to a host or hosts, and to their offspring before dying.

Over decades, insects and arthropods have developed resistance to insecticide formulas. Therefore scientists are designing increasingly complex formulas to eliminate ticks and other pests. Some of the surprising toxins and microbes that have been or may be added to insecticide formulas include scorpion, sea urchin, spider, and frog toxins; human proteins (genes); plant and insect viruses, and even serious past human health threats, such as *bubonic plague.*[13,16,18-23,195]

When patients present with symptoms after a tick bite, physicians should consider whether to check for other tick-transmitted infections (co-infections). Multiple infections are commonly seen with tickborne illness. These infections seem to vary by geographic region. Some of the more commonly detected infections include these; some of which live inside of cells (*intracellular*).

- *Human Monocytic* or *Granulocytic Ehrlichiosis* (HME/HGE)
- *Bartonella henselae, Afipia felis,* and other bartonella and afipia strains which cause human cat scratch fevers[161,162]
- *Anaplasma phagocytophilum*
- *Giardia species*
- *Leptospires* and *Leptonemas* (I cover these agents in a separate section)
- *Microsporidia, Sporozoa, Piroplasms,* other protists including *Coccidians*:
    - *Babesia* (Malaria-like, common strains: *B. duncani, B. microti, B. divergens*)
    - *Cryptosporidium*
    - *Cyclospora*
    - *Isospora*
    - *Toxoplasma gondii*
    - *Protomyxzoa rheumatica* (*FL1953*)
- *Theileria microti* and other species (livestock infections, f/k/a *Babesia microti*)
- *Chlamydia pneumonia* (surprisingly common in Lyme patients)
- Rocky Mountain spotted fever (*Rickettsia rickettsii*)
- *Mycoplasmas* (especially strains *M. pneumonia, hominis, fermentans, penetrans*)
- *Pseudomonas* species (*P. fluorescens, P. aeruginosa*)
- Spiroplasmas (covered in a separate section, these are mycoplasma "parents")

- Tickborne relapsing fevers (many species which may be part of a Bb agent)
- Tick paralysis
- STARI (Southern Tick-Associated Rash Illness) or *Borrelia lonestari*
- *Borrelia miyamotoi, B. andersonii, B. japonica* or other Lyme-like infections that are more closely related to tickborne relapsing fevers than to Bb. This may mean they lack a key component of a mutated Bb spirochete (i.e. the spiroplasma or leptonema portion).
- Tularemia (rabbit or deer fly fever)
- Brucella strains (Malta fever, Brucellosis, Bang's disease)
- Q-Fever (*Coxiella burnetii*)
- *Helicobactor pylori*
- *Clostridia* species
- *Legionella* species

Other infections are common to Lyme-transmitting ticks, including regionally-dependent parasites, fungi and viruses. The following *viruses* have been isolated from Lyme-transmitting ticks around the world.

- Rubivirus (*Rubella* virus)
- Powassan (deer tick) virus
- Tickborne encephalitis
- Russian Spring-Summer encephalitis (RSSE)
- Australian X (Murray Valley encephalitis)
- California group viruses (commonly found in ticks)
- Corona viruses (i.e. Runde virus of seabird ticks) *which cause persistent infections*
- Reoviruses (insect and plant viruses commonly found in ticks)
- Poxviruses (i.e. mousepox; a latent virus in wild and lab mouse populations)
- Rabies (related to most of the aforementioned viruses)
- *Lone Star* virus (Strain "TMA 1381" first isolated from Lone Star ticks [*Amblyomma Americanum*] in 1966-1967).
- Any of a number of plant and insect viruses and bacteriae[13-16]

Tickborne infections may include a tick-transmitted *Arbovirus* ("Arbo" = Arthropod-borne). Each virus listed above is a tick-transmissible arbovirus. Some of these viruses have never been considered to be part of tickborne infections, and yet viruses appear to be an important aspect. Arboviruses produce symptoms that are similar to those of Lyme disease, including fever, fatigue, rashes, encephalitis, conjunctivitis, adenopathies, and arthralgias. The difference between Lyme disease and arbovirus infections are said not always to be plainly evident. Some symptoms of "Lyme" may be coming from an arbovirus portion of a tickborne infection.[48]

There seems to be a *tick-transmitted virus* at the heart of some or all Lyme disease, STARI, Morgellons, or other tickborne infections. This is important because research shows that Bb spirochetes have a resident virus. It is a *bacteriophage* (virus that infects bacteria). A virus explains the relapsing/remitting symptoms of Lyme and related infections, especially where spirochetes or their virus-infected remnants persist. Virus type could certainly create differences between Lyme borrelia and dissimilar borrelia (i.e. *B. lonestari, B. miyamotoi, B. andersonii*).[165,169]

Viral Reactivation

Tickborne infections are complicated by the landscape of the human body. Important human viruses are commonly detected in tickborne infection patients. These include *Epstein-barr* virus (EBV), *Cytomegalovirus* (CMV), and/or human *Herpes* viruses (HHV-1, HHV-2, HHV-6, HHV-7).

Tickborne infections complicate a heavily burdened human immune system. Most people carry a lifetime of exposures to natural infections, vaccines, chemicals, heavy metals, and other toxins. When confronted with the addition of tickborne infections, the body is unable to properly defend itself. We may wonder from where have some of these viruses come? Some are a result of past infections, while others are transmitted by a tick which previously fed upon a reptile, bird, or other animal.

We already know that latent infections can come back to life inside a tick body under stress. Likewise when our bodies are stressed, latent viruses can also reactivate. The reactivation of latent viruses also occurs in wild and laboratory mouse populations. Mice are an important host to ticks and to Lyme bacteria.[13,16,42]

Several *herpes* virus strains are frequently found in Lyme patients. One such virus is *Roseola infantum*, the human herpes virus 6 (HHV-6). Herpes viruses are also commonly found in ticks. Roseola is a relatively mild viral infection that most people had in childhood. Some people are now positive for the virus after a tick bite. Active HHV-6 can cause encephalitis, pneumonia, and bone marrow problems.[170]

I found a description of an EM-like rash called *Roseola annulata* in an old medical textbook. This rash is oddly similar to the bull's-eye rash of Lyme disease. Roseola is also called sixth disease, rose rash, or *Pseudorubella.* Here is a description of the *Roseola annulata* rash from my 1857 textbook:[13,16,17]

> *"On the lower extremities, and sometimes on other parts, we observe several rose-coloured rings, varying in diameter from a quarter of an inch to an inch. The colour of the skin within the rings is quite natural...several diseases of the skin have the same tendency to affect a ring-shape, the part within the ring being, in all respects, healthy."*

This kind of rash certainly appears to resemble a Lyme bull's-eye rash. The source says that a roseola infection may last from days to several weeks. This period is consistent with the display, expansion, and disappearance of a Lyme bull's-eye rash. While a past natural roseola infection might provide protection against another human roseola virus, it may not protect us from an insect, animal, or yeast virus from the same, or a compatible family to which we have no natural immunity.

The source also describes the constitutional symptoms found with this human form of roseola/pseudo-rubella. They are similar to the "flu-like" symptoms found during acute Lyme disease, or those caused by an arbovirus. Are Lyme rashes caused by a tick-transmitted virus?[49-51]

Reoviruses are also found in ticks that transmit Lyme disease. Reoviruses can infect bacteria. They also infect fungi and yeasts that are important to the tickborne infection story. In humans, reoviruses cause gut and respiratory problems. The human viruses of tickborne infection patients can reactivate. The added burden of tickborne infections weakens the immune system. If sleeping human viruses are reawakened into active states just as they are in insects, then people with tickborne illnesses may benefit from anti-virals or other therapies to address these reactivations.[49-51]

Yeasts, Fungi, and Tickborne Infections

There are various *fungi, yeasts,* and environmental *molds* that are found in the areas where ticks live. These pathogens are found upon and within tick bodies because of contact exposures. These pathogens certainly may play an active role in tickborne illness. Some of the most common fungi include those found in forests and in microbial insecticides. When wild yeast or fungal strains intermix, they can create toxic strains. While antibiotics are useful against tickborne illnesses, anti-fungals and agents to address yeasts have proven to be additionally helpful.[13,16]

Fungi that are infectious to ticks and insects are called *entomopathogenic.* These fungi typically produce *Aflatoxins* that are highly neurotoxic to humans. Some fungal strains are pathogenic (infectious), while others are not (*saprophytes*). But the saprophytes can become pathogenic if they become virus-infected or if they mix with toxic strains.[25]

Reoviruses can also infect fungi (i.e. chestnut blight fungus *Cryphonectria parasitica*). Chestnut blight is an important global forest fungus of chestnut trees. Oaks are another species often infected with wild yeasts (i.e. *Saccharomyces paradoxus*) and infectious fungi (i.e. *Mycotypha indica*). *Oak wilt* is another fungus (*Endoconidiophora fagacearum n/k/a Ceratocystis fagacearum*), but any tree fungus can infect ticks.[171-181,197,198]

Oak wilt is common among oaks throughout the world. Trees are important to the tickborne infection story since insect larvae and animals (i.e. moths, mice, deer) feed upon trees and their nuts. Animals are important hosts to Lyme bacteria and other tickborne infections. Tick-transmissible viruses that infect fungi are closely related to tick, mouse, deer, and human viruses (i.e. Colorado tick fever, Eyach). Some of the reoviruses have been isolated from Lyme disease patients.[62-64]

Ticks transmit yeast and fungi to humans on contact, or when feeding. This is why physicians might consider therapies which treat regionally important forest fungi and yeasts in their tickborne illness patients. It is also why it may be important to remediate fungal or yeast toxins which cause neurotoxin-related symptoms. The following fungi have been detected in and upon Lyme-transmitting ticks. The first seven are also known to be used as insecticides around the world.[196]

- *Aspergillus flavus* (fungi of cereal crops, legumes)
- *Beauveria bassiana**
- *Isaria* species
- *Entomophthora*
- *Lecanicillium* species (found in Connecticut and New York ticks)
- *Metarhizium anisopliae* and *M. flavoviride* strains†
- *Paecilomyces fumosoroseus* (and other species)
- *Spicaria rileyi*
- *Sporotrichum globuliferum* (found in the midwestern United States)
- *Verticillium*

**Used as an insecticide since the 1850's in Europe, and 1867 in the US. One of the most common fungi used.*
†This fungus was launched in South Africa in 1998 and in other areas including Western Africa in later years. It is a commonly used fungal insecticide around the world.

The next list includes fungi known to be pathogenic to ticks; and that were isolated from them. It is impossible to know what kind of fungi or yeasts a tick may carry. Any applied or natural fungi/yeasts could become part of tickborne infections. Some physicians use broad spectrum anti-fungals during tickborne infection treatments to address fungal infections.

Aspergillus flavus	*Blastomyces*	*Candida*
Chlamydia	*Coccidiodes immitus*	*Coelomomyces*
Conidiobolus	*Cordyceps*	*Cryptococcus*
Entomophaga	*Entomophthora*	*Erynia*
Fungi imperfecti	*Fusarium*	*Hirsutella*
Histoplasma	*Kluyveromyces lactis*	*Lagenidium*
Lecanicillium lecanii	*Leptographia*	*Microascus brevicaulis*
Nomuraea	*Nosema**	*Pandora*
Penicillium	*Simplicillium lamellicola*	*Scopulariopsis brevicaulis*
Tichothecium	*Tolypocladium*	*Zoophthore*[13,16,24,25,43]

**Nosema are microsporidia that were reclassified as fungi.*

Like little trojan horses, fungal infections carried by ticks can also harbor their own co-infections (i.e. yeast, mold, viruses, bacteria). For example, the insecticide fungus *Beauveria bassiana* has its own parasite; a fungi called *Melanospora parasitica.* Fungi are commonly virus-infected.

Wild yeasts and fungi are important to think about since they may adversely interact with the yeasts and other microbes found within commercial microbial insecticides. The interactions between insecticidal microbes and whatever else ticks pick up from the environment may play a role in tickborne infections. In the soil and inside the tick gut, microbes may shuffle and mix (reassort) their genes to create mutant or toxic strains which may be passed to humans through a tick bite or other tick exposures.

How do we fix the problem of toxic yeast strains if they exist in our bodies? Remember that we have natural yeasts which live in our body including *Candida albicans.* We should think about replenishing the gut using healthy brewer's yeast (*Saccharomyces cerevisiae*) and other probiotics. Physicians may also need to eliminate unhealthy gut bacteria such as the opportunistic human *Flavobacterium, Weeksella virosa.*[13,16]

Like insects and arthropods, our gut bacteriae become infected by the microbes found in the foods we eat; from our environment, and from the infections to which we are exposed. Lyme treating physicians are wise who promote the use of various high-quality probiotics. These can help to restore gut flora to healthy levels after they have become altered by infections, a poor diet, and/or the use of antibiotics.

Physicians do not have the time nor ability to screen patients for every known tick pathogen. However, they might assess patients based on symptom presentation and known regional pathogens. It certainly helps to learn of the kinds of pathogens which lurk upon and within a tick body. While no one wishes to imagine how many transmissible infections are found inside a particular tick, it is important for physicians not to take a "one size fits all" approach to treating patients who have tickborne infections. Each person's *infection complex* is as unique as the infected individual; as well as the tiny tick (or insect) that bit them.[13,16]

What in the World is Wolbachia?

There are other highly important tick-transmissible pathogens that may become part of tickborne infections. Ticks carry a number of fungi, microsporidiae, protozoae, flukes, nematodes (worms), other parasites, and their *symbiont organisms*. One of the most important and common tickborne parasites are *nematodes.* These are microscopic to visually detectable worms (*filaria* or *helminths*). These micro-sized worms also carry an important human infection from their *symbiont* organism.

A symbiont organism is an infectious parasite that lives inside the body of another organism. Ticks are commonly infected with nematodes. A symbiont organism that nematodes *require* in order for them to be able to reproduce is a tiny intracellular infection called *Wolbachia.*[13,16]

Wolbachia is a reproductive bacterial parasite of nematodes, insects, arthropods, animals, and humans. Wolbachia may contribute to human infertility. Treatment of *Wolbachia* infections includes the use of a tetracycline (i.e. doxycycline). Patients with tickborne infections that include nematodes, show improvement after treatment with drugs which target the worms (anti-helminthics). Doxycycline is usually prescribed for Lyme disease. It may have a dual benefit in that it kills wolbachia infections in patients who are co-infected with tick nematodes.

Nematodes can burrow within the soft tissues of the eyes. Research papers reveal that a massive killing of nematodes may contribute to a loss of vision. They discuss an alternative method of removing nematodes using doxycycline. The drug does not effectively kill the nematodes, but it does kill their wolbachia symbiont. Without wolbachia, the nematodes cannot reproduce. Thus they die at the end of their life cycle, preserving delicate eye tissues from the effects of a rapid nematodal die-off.[13,16,44,45]

Silent Partners

Ticks also transmit important *Flavobacteria.* I believe that bacteria from the *Cytophaga-Flavobacterium* group are an important aspect of tickborne infections. This group contains tiny insect virus-infected bacteriae which cause diseases in ticks and in crop and forestry insects.

Such pests include but are not limited to cabbage, armyworm, silkworm, gypsy, and other moth larvae; Japanese and other beetle larvae, and other insects and arthropods. These bacteriae also commonly infect the wasps and mites which parasitize ticks. Bacteria are often co-infected with intracellular viruses which normally lie *latent.* Latent viruses can reactivate in the presence of stressors including radiation, insecticides, and chemicals.

Tiny sawfly insect *baculoviruses* (i.e. *borrelina viruses*) have been released by scientists to accelerate the effects of microbial insecticides. These releases began in Connecticut during the 1950's, shortly before the discovery of odd, mutated spirochetes and the Connecticut outbreak of human Lyme disease. Immediately after field trials were undertaken, techniques on cultivating tiny insect viruses and samples of same were offered globally to interested laboratories for insecticidal use.[103-105]

The insect baculoviruses that were released work in tandem with a group of soil-borne bacteria called *Extremophiles.* This is a group of microbes which thrive under extreme conditions. Extremophiles are very difficult to kill. Some species live in high or low temperatures, and others cannot be killed even in outer space or with nuclear radiation. The baculoviruses have an affinity not only for soil bacteria, but also for arthropods including ticks. When baculoviruses and soil bacteria are combined, they work together as more powerful infective agents. My concern is over their safety including the possible extension of their natural host range due to their global presence and repeated use within or in addition to microbial insecticides.[103-105,115]

Extremophiles produce enzymes which break down agricultural and other chemicals, nuclear wastes, industrial pollutants, and microbial insecticides. This may help GM microbes mix with, contaminate, and become contaminated by environmental microbes to which ticks and other blood feeders are likewise exposed.[13,16]

Some of the insect and arthropod diseases caused by bacteria that are virally-infected (*phages*),* produce peculiar color-changing effects in insect larvae such as silkworm and Japanese beetle larvae (i.e. "black," "blue," "reds," or "milky spore" infections discussed in two of my books).[13,16]

**Phages are tiny viruses that infect bacteria. Baculoviruses are phages.*

The Bb bacterium was found to have a *phage* virus. I believe that when examined closely, Bb strains will reveal the presence of important insect viruses and bacteria, including some which cannot easily be detected upon culture. Insects that are sick with some of these bacteria/virus combinations can only be diagnosed much like the way that Lyme patients are – on the basis of physical symptoms. This is because these infections cannot be cultured in a laboratory except with highly specialized techniques. There are no commercial laboratory tests to detect most of the extremophile agents if they make their way into our bodies.[13,16,100-102]

However there are a few patents which describe how to detect borrelia and extremophiles (in particular sulfur-reducing bacteria and their extremophile viruses) from wastewaters or from urine. Some of these bacteria are natural. Others are genetically engineered to be copper and metal tolerant to leach metals from ores; for oil/gas/mineral wellbores (in situ mining), or to bioremediate acid mine and radioactive nuclear wastes.* Extremophiles are unique as they have multiple copies of genes in each cell. This allows them to persist under extreme conditions (or in the presence of antibiotics). Industrially and agriculturally important organic compounds called "Tweens" significantly increase their growth.[184-187]

*The first human cluster of Lyme disease emerged in Connecticut, a state with a rich copper mining history.

Research shows that the introduction of soil bacteria (*Bacillus ce-*

reus) to cultures of *Cytophaga-Flavobacteria* bacteria (CF) helps these extremophiles grow. The globally-used insecticide *Bacillus thuringiensis* (B.t.) is a close relative of *Bacillus cereus* and *Bacillus anthracis* (anthrax). These soil bacteriae are extremophiles, and so are some of the insect viruses mentioned earlier. This tells us that exposures to these microbes may cause infections that are difficult to detect, and also to treat.[100,101]

Soils where B.t. is used may contain a higher concentration of the extremophiles, including the CF group of bacteria and their phage viruses. Agricultural and industrial insecticides are often accompanied by chemical fertilizers. These also help certain strains of bacteria, fungi, and viruses thrive since they alter soil nutrients (i.e. increase manganese content). Bb bacteria thrive in manganese-rich environments including in soils and watersheds into which soils drain; but then again so do the other microbes which live in, and upon blood feeding insects and arthropods.[106-108]

GM insecticides also use *polyhedrosis* (polygonol) and *granulosis* (granular) insect baculoviruses. Important phage baculoviruses of insecticides include *Autographa californica, Galleria mellonella, Heliothis zea, Trichoplusia ni,* and others. These viruses are also found in naturally infected insects (i.e. moths, sawflies) and arthropods as *latent infections*. Phage viruses including the baculoviruses can "lyse" or open up spirochetes to infect them.[123-128]

The African *Sindbis* virus has also been used extensively, including to genetically engineer fall armyworm larvae (Sf 9) cells to produce (express) baculovirus genes for insecticides. Sindbis virus is felt to be the parent virus of most, if not every encephalitis-causing insect/arthropod arbovirus. Bb bacteria appear to have an infectious insect arbovirus/phage component.

It is yet unproven if genes from insecticide-exposed insects make their way into the human body through tick inoculation. It is well-known that insects harbor soil bacteria, fungi, and viruses. What insects ingest and contact mutates within their gut to create new, transmissible infections.

Natural microbes and those from insecticides are assisted in gene-swapping processes by agricultural and industrial chemicals. These make their way into soils and watersheds; in particular to wastewater plants. We already know that insecticides are meant to reactivate infections inside the bodies of insects and arthropods. We do not however yet know if they may be able to behave similarly inside the human body after tick inoculation. We are just beginning to learn which microbes thrive inside the bodies of ticks. Insect inoculations are just the obvious way that microbes of diseases like Lyme or Morgellons enter our bodies. Other less apparent routes may include food, or by wastewater that has been inadequately treated.[129-133]

Anthrax and anthrax-related soil bacteria are in the environment. Related species are found at considerably higher levels in recent decades due to the use of microbial insecticides. We might consider whether a fermentable soil bacteria can cause or contribute to tickborne, or to on-contact human infections. Anthrax spores survive in soils for hundreds of years. There is a skin (cutaneous) form of anthrax called "wool sorter's disease." This is an anthrax infection which causes ulcerative skin lesions. The lesions look strikingly similar to those seen upon Morgellons patients (in terms of ulceration and scarring characteristics).

A textbook which served as an early guidebook for insecticide design describes how *Bacillus anthracis* (anthrax) spores are fermentable under certain temperatures in a neutralized bouillon for twenty days. This downgrades their toxins to a weakened, less infectious state.[111]

Sheep and other grazing animals may ingest natural anthrax spores and other soil bacteria when they graze. In the sheep gut, anthrax spores undergo a natural fermentation process where they become infectious. What if a similar process occurs in insects or mammals that are exposed to anthrax-related soil bacteria? Could humans be exposed to an "almost" anthrax by a tick inoculation of microbes that were contaminated by natural or man-made insecticide formulas? Could an infected soil spirochete cause a very Lyme-like cutaneous anthrax disease called Morgellons?[111]

Does Morgellons Exist?

A group of patients have turned up since the late 1990's with an odd illness and symptoms which often resemble Lyme disease. There are several names that have been assigned to the disorder, including neuro-cutaneous syndrome, delusional parasitosis, and Morgellons. At first glance, the so-called Morgellons disease appears to be a more complex version of Lyme disease. Morgellons constitutional symptoms are similar to those of Lyme; but with the additional burden of strange multi-colored "fibers" or hairs which appear to grow from unsightly skin lesions. These lesions are not seen with "typical" Lyme disease; and not all patients with Morgellons may have a Bb infection.[87-95]

An American named Mary Leitao was credited with the first report of Morgellons in 2001, when she noticed that an ulcerative lesion on her two-year old son's lip produced strange fibers or hairs. The name Morgellons disease was coined by Mary after finding a description of what she thought was a similar illness in a 15th-century French publication.[93-95]

Only recently has anyone said to have cultured a borrelia strain from a Morgellons patient's lesion. For years Lyme physicians have been treating

Morgellons patients aggressively using antibiotics which target borrelia strains. These antibiotics resolve many Morgellons patient's symptoms, including the strange fiber-producing lesions. Only some of the more advanced cases do not seem to respond to antibiotics.[96]

In several of my earlier books I described Morgellons as a "Lyme-plus" infection. It is the "plus" part that concerns me. I also describe the history of genetically modified organisms including formulas that use genes from the bacteria *Agrobacterium tumefaciens*; as well as important insect viruses. This bacterium causes tumors (galls) to grow on infected plants. According to my research, Bb strains appear to have fungal, viral, spirochetal, and other components. An environmentally-acquired infection is not difficult to assume. Scientists have isolated *A. tumefaciens* from some Morgellons patients, but not from others.[13,16,97]

Other scientists have concluded that this bacteria is not the cause of Morgellons when they could not culture *A. tumefaciens* from patient samples. This may mean that the patients were not infected with the bacteria. But the ability to culture an agent is not always possible. It can remain latent; and only fractions of the organism may be required to swap genes (*horizontally transfer*) between plants and perhaps insects or animals.

Agrobacterium tumefaciens is a natural bacterium. It is also a frequently used bacterial vehicle in the genetic laboratory for plant cultivation, for applied insecticides, and for plant-based insect resistance. The use of only a few genes in an *expression cassette* are necessary to manually infect plant cells. There may not be enough genetic material available to detect by any laboratory means in infected insect or other samples.

Other organisms used in the lab to transfer genes for GM products are *Pichia pastoria, Escherichia coli* (*E. coli*), and *Pseudomonas aeruginosa.* The first is a fermentable fungus that can be used with brewer's yeast

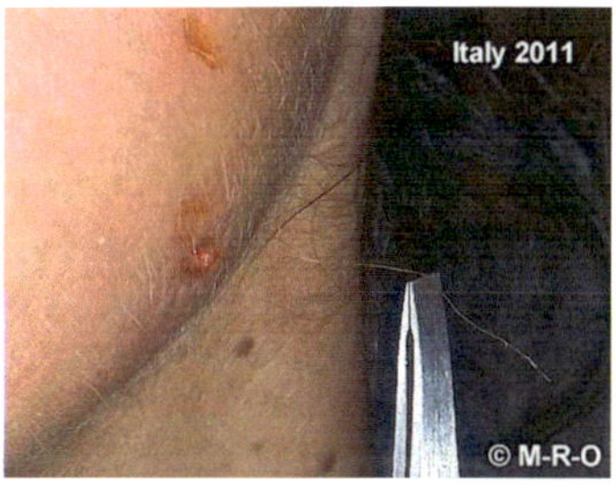

Morgellons lesions. Photos courtesy Marc Neuman, Augsburg, Germany.

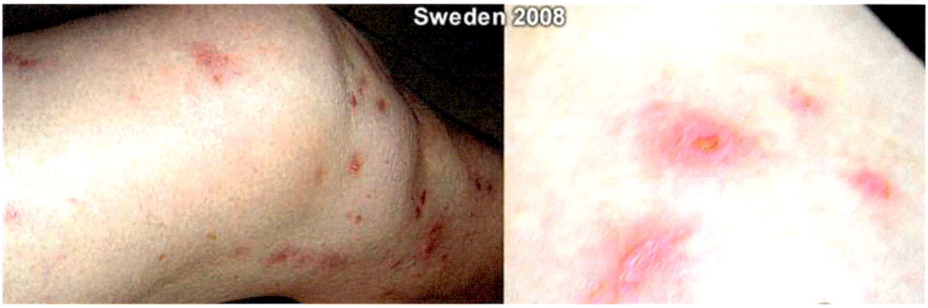

(*Saccharomyces cerevisiae*); for example to ferment microbial insecticides during the manufacturing process. The last is an opportunistic bacterium; and one that is used to bioremediate chemical and nuclear wastes. It can also be contracted from contaminated surgical products. Some people have expressed concerns over accidental GM gene transfers between plants through cross-pollination; or the accidental transfer of GM formulas by diet or insect inoculation to higher mammals.[99]

A problem with some of these agents (i.e. *Pseudomonas*) is an ability to swap genes with other microbes. For example, it is easy to find other bacteria in a hospital setting, such as *Methicillin-resistant Staphylococcus aureus* (MRSA), or (plain) *Staphylococcus.* Both microbes can create flesh "eating" lesions. Either may mutate with fungi or other bacteria to cause a Morgellons-like infection in co-infected patients.

Like the silkworm diseases that change the color of larval silk to red, black, blue, and other hues; the peculiar hair-like fibers found among Morgellons skin lesions produce similar colors. Such hues can be made by keratin, the fibrous protein substance in the body that produces our skin, hair, and nails. Human vellus and other hair can become structurally altered during tickborne and other infections. The exact composition of Morgellons fibers are unknown. Keratin and collagen breaks down during tickborne infections. Morgellons hair-like fibers continue to grow, do not always come from hair follicles, and are often painful to remove.

Just like Lyme patients, people with Morgellons have been called crazy, and have at times been diagnosed with delusional parasitosis. Perhaps insect virus-infected, fungi-like bacteria are at the root of the skin manifestations of Morgellons. The question of course is whether the infective cocktail accidentally contains lab-manipulated genes or is simply a happenstance of the microbes in a tick gut or other environmental exposure.

The recent discovery of a Bb strain from a Morgellons patient skin culture does not necessarily mean that Morgellons lesions are caused by a Bb infection. However it does lend credence that Morgellons has an infectious source which may at least sometimes include a Bb spirochete.[116]

If a Bb spirochete is infected with the same agents found in a Morgellons patient who does not have Bb, the outcome may be similar. Both may produce symptoms of Morgellons; only the Lyme-plus patient will have an additional spirochetal infection. This may be why some of the same chemotherapies used in Lyme treatment help many Morgellons patients. Some of the persistent infections may be due to the presence of an extremophile organism. According to research, therapies for extremophile bacteria may include Beta-lactam agents (i.e. imipenem or cefuroxime [ceftin]).[116]

What has also not yet been discussed in the Morgellons arena is a *Flavobacterium* that is known to cause a disease in fish; "cotton-wool" disease. The agent responsible for this infection is *Flavobacterium columnare* (it has several names). It was thought to be a fungus, but it is a bacteria. There are also slime molds and other molds found in fish and water, along the lines of *Saprolegnia* and *Achlya* which produce a white cottony appearance on infected fish.

The molds, viruses, and bacteria found in fresh and oceanic waters are important not only because ticks thrive in these environments. They are important since migratory birds eat a marine diet; and patients with Morgellons presentations are typically found along coastal areas and other waterways where marine birds and their ticks live.

A fungal/viral/bacterial agent and rampant or "runaway" genes may explain Morgellons lesions and their hairs or other artifacts that are not produced by spirochetes. Lesions may be from tick or insect inoculation; environmental exposure (i.e. airborne, contact); or contaminated foods. Insect viruses infect bacteria and fungi. Insecticides wash into waterways adjacent to tick habitats. Insecticides contain a large group of GM virus, bacteria, fungi; and insect, animal, or human genes. If microbial enzymes disrupt the structure of insecticidal formulas, anything is possible.[13,16]

When I began researching my book *God Science* in 2009, I studied the diseases of silkworm moth and Japanese beetle larvae. I was interested in learning how infections cause silk and insect body colors to change to yellow, red, blue, or black pigments. It seemed curious that the fibers found in Morgellons skin lesions appear in a similar color range. I suspected that skin pigment genes were triggered during insect infections.[16]

Could the colored Morgellons fibers be caused by virus-led gene activity in skin cells? Is this driven by a hair pigment-altering, insect virus-infected bacteria that mutated with a fungus? Are the lesions nothing more than fungi superinfected with *Pseudomonas aeruginosa,* or *Staphylococcus* (strep) bacteria, and that are antibiotic-resistant in some patients? Multi-tiered infections are found in nature, and they are also created in the lab for insecticide, pharmaceutical, and industrial products. These agents are also found in hospital settings and in polluted and treated wastewaters where they thrive (i.e. *Pseudomonas, E. coli,* or *Flavobacterium* strains).[188]

Scientists also manipulate genes from silk-producing spiders and mites, and pigmented bacteria and fungi. Infectious agents could supply human skin cells with the "wrong" genetic information, similar to what occurs in infected silkworm moth larvae. Perhaps Morgellons patients are infected with a bacteria or fungus that is super infected with a pigment-altering

The Lesions of Morgellons

All but one of these images (marked) are photos of Morgellons lesions or artifacts from such lesions. The exception is the photo of infectious impetigo. Are Morgellons lesions caused by a mutated *Pseudomonas* or other fungi that is super infected with a virus and an antibiotic-resistant bacteria (i.e. strep/staph)? If so, some Bb strains could harbor this infectious cocktail or it could be a tickborne co-infection. Morgellons could simply be a contact infection that is not tickborne.

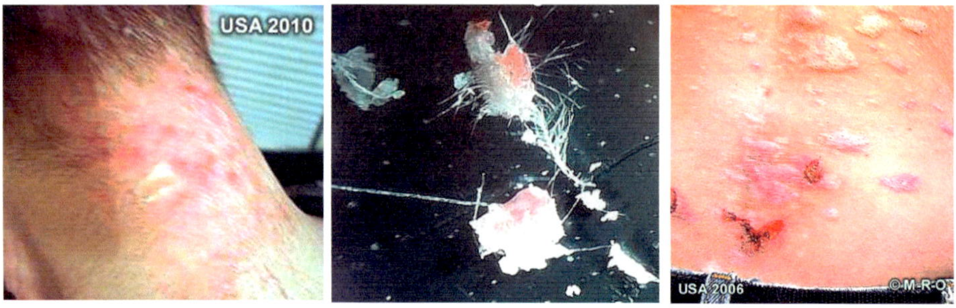

The skin lesions of Morgellons patients are painful and disfiguring. The wounds are slow to heal, and "fibers," hairs, or other strange artifacts can be recovered from them. Some wounds are devastating.

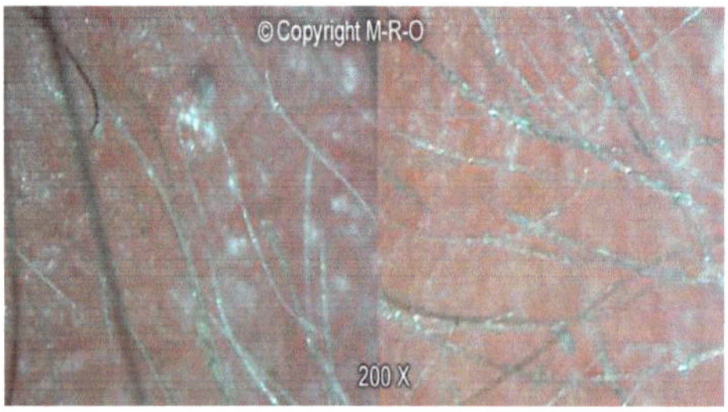

Above: 200X magnification of some of the transparent hairs. Below: Skin sloughing and shedding found in some Morgellons cases.

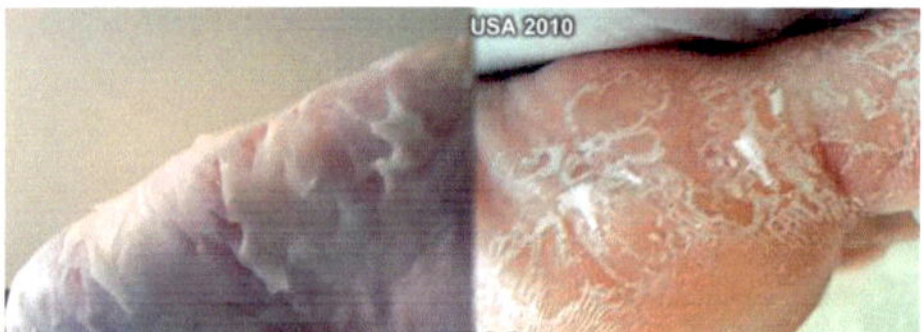

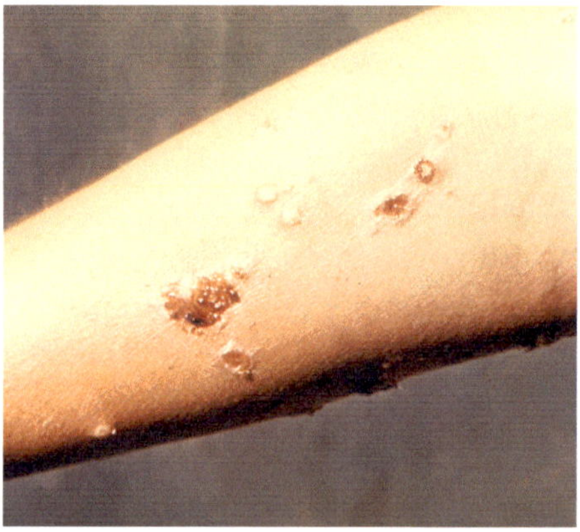

Above: Lesions of a *Streptococcal* impetigo infection. This is often caused by a *Staphylococcus aureus* bacteria. Its lesions are similar to those seen on Morgellons patients. The infection is spread by contact, including by linens and clothing. CDC photo.

Below, 160X magnification. Strange colored fibers. "Fibers" can be yellow, white, transparent, blue, black, red, or orange. They often contain cottony or gelatinous bleb or biofilm-like attachments. Some patients have insect infestations (i.e. collembola, demodex mites). A few patients claim to have removed insect parts from some of their lesions. A few patients first noticed the illness after surgery; not from a perceptible insect bite. *All unmarked photos: Marc Neuman, Augsburg Germany.*

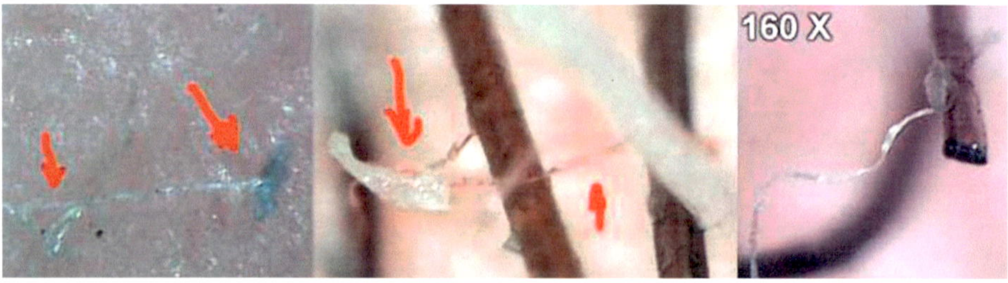

insect virus. Such infections could produce the wounds, fibers, cottony growths, and other artifacts found upon Morgellons patients' skin.[129-133]

Tick or insect inoculation may be only one transmission route for a disease like Morgellons. Another route may include the ingestion of foods that are contaminated with microbial insecticides. Scientists and their studies discuss the safety of microbial insecticides; and claim that these microbes pass through the human digestive tract without harm, although independent research seems to suggest otherwise.[19,20,23]

A third route of contamination by a Morgellons agent may be surgical. Some patients have complained of this disorder only after having surgery. Infections can be spread surgically. We may also suspect sterilized water solutions or surgical products (i.e. human albumin).[119-121,159]

These products were found to have been contaminated with microbes that are important to tickborne infection history. A 1977 paper co-authored by Rheumatologist Allen C. Steere discussed the earlier contamination of human albumin with *Pseudomonas aeruginosa* and other *Pseudomonas* species. Wastewaters contain spirochetes and important extremophile bacteria that are not easily removed from commercial or residential water supplies.[119-121,159,161]

A novel therapy is felt to activate the *Alternative Cellular Energy* (ACE) pathway in skin to treat various "stealth" viruses including herpes. It involves the use of moringa oil or neutral red pigment and UV light to activate these pathways and to aid the healing process. Lyme and Morgellons patients are likely to have active herpes and other viruses which affect skin cells (i.e. herpes causes skin lesions).[109,110]

The agent that causes Morgellons is still unknown. Perhaps it is caused by mutated or "downgraded" anthrax-like bacteria; or more simply, opportunistic virus-infected bacteria and/or fungi. The obvious cause of Morgellons is an infection. The antibiotic Ciprofloxacin (Cipro) is the first line of defense for cutaneous anthrax. Some physicians are beginning to treat their Lyme and Morgellons patients using this antibiotic.

Spiroplasmas and Leptonemas

I believe that two of the most intriguing pieces of the tickborne infection puzzle have had no practical discussion in the medical arena outside of my published books – *Spiroplasmas* and *Leptonemas*. Because these agents have been isolated from ticks and from Lyme patients, it is important to include them in our tickborne infection discussion.

Spiroplasmas

The smallest group of self-replicating organisms known to exist include plant and animal bacteriae that lack a cell wall (wall-less); the *Mollicutes*. These bacteriae are part of a larger group of *Mycoplasmatales*. *Mycoplasmas* are typically found as co-infections in Lyme patients, and this is important since *Mycoplasmas* are degraded (genetically reduced) *Spiroplasma* forms. *Spiroplasmas* are the cause of the "yellows" diseases of plants that are found in nutrient-altered soils. Spiroplasma/mycoplasma infections are very difficult to treat. They are commonly resistant to penicillins, rifampicins, and tetracyclines. They also easily mutate, making them quickly resistant to other antibiotics.[76,77,160]

The mollicute group includes a large number of *spiroplasma* strains. Spiroplasma infections may be related to human *yellow fever*. This infection is caused partly by a tick or mosquito-transmitted arbovirus from the same group that cause encephalitis; but it may also have a spiroplasma component. The arbovirus group includes viruses that are used to make human vaccines; and also a wild-type *Rubella* virus.

Spiroplasmas and their smaller mycoplasma forms harbor parasitic phage viruses or *Virus-Like Particles* (VLP). I wrote extensively about important insect and plant viruses in two of my books. Spiroplasmas change forms (pleomorphic) as Bb spirochetes do. Spiroplasmas and Bb have a cholesterol-like membrane and appear to be related to *Clostridia* bacteria; a group that includes *Tetanus* and *Botulism* (food poisoning).[13,16,78,79]

Just like Bb, spiroplasmas are tough to culture in the laboratory. They are known to cause ocular (eye), urogenital, arthritic, brain, and neurologic disease in mammals. Also like Bb, spiroplasmas live in magnesium and manganese-rich environments. Spiroplasma-infected plants show symptoms of magnesium deficiency similar to that found in Lyme patients.

Like Bb, spiroplasmas produce cell wall-less, spherical, spiral (helical), non-spiral, bleb, gemma, and motile (moving) forms. Spiroplasmas change shape the way Bb does; by casting off outer proteins and other structures when challenged environmentally or chemically. Spiroplasmas produce key proteins that are detectable in the 25 to 30-kDa* range. This is the same range that some lab tests report for Bb spirochetes.[58-61]

**kDa refers to kilodalton, a molecular unit of measure by which antibodies are recorded, and which appear on some laboratory tests as banding patterns.*

Spiroplasma spirochetes appear identical to Bb under dark field microscropy (a visualization technique). The two spirochetes may be mistaken one for the other. Spiroplasmas are detectable using broad-range PCR-TTGE testing (temporal temperature gradient gel electrophoresis). Some public health experts claim that PCR testing for Bb is unreliable. However it makes sense that PCR would be useful since research suggests that Bb has a spiroplasma component.[13,16,58-61]

Spiroplasmas were once in the same category as a swine gut infection called *"swine flu."* This is interesting since two mollicute strains known to cause knee arthritis in pigs are *Mycoplasma hyorhinis* and *Mycoplasma Hyosynoviae.* Lyme patients have mycoplasma infections which can produce joint arthritis, particularly in the large joints including the knees.

The largest spiroplasma is the tick *Spiroplasma ixodetis Y32.* Research suggests that spiroplasma spirochetes may be killed by preventing their escape from the "lag phase" of their growth cycle. There may be antibiotics which attack the organisms during this phase.[52-54]

Spiroplasmas were first discovered in 1944 in citrus trees as citrus "stubborn" disease. Two decades later Dr. Willy Burgdorfer (the scientist after whom the Lyme disease spirochete was named) and colleagues isolated a new spiroplasma from rabbit ticks. It was felt to be similar to citrus tree spiroplasmas. They named it the "277F" agent.[62,78,79]

Dr. Burgdorfer has classified the 277F agent in the category of *Actinomycetes.* This is a spore-forming, thread-like filamentous soil bacteria that is spirochetal in form (a fungi-like bacteria).[114]

Before and during the mid-1970's when a new arthritis outbreak appeared in Connecticut (Lyme disease), Dr. Burgdorfer and colleagues where intently studying the spiroplasmas. A spiroplasma connection may be why the Bb spirochete was named after Dr. Burgdorfer.[62-64,75]

In 1981, the year the Lyme disease "agent" was identified, a brand new spiroplasma was isolated from Oregon western black-legged ticks *Ixodes pacificus*. These ticks are important transmitters of human Lyme disease and other tickborne infections. Tick symbionts were being studied by National Institutes of Health scientists including Dr. Burgdorfer decades before, and during the early Connecticut outbreak of Lyme disease; before Bb was announced to the world.[62,65,72,73,80]

The new Oregon tick spiroplasma was isolated from ticks collected between December 1979 and July 1980. The tick cultures were incubated for about three weeks before spiroplasmas could be isolated. This is similar to the culture-type tests for human Lyme disease. They require a long incubation period to detect slow-growing spirochetes. Antibody tests are favored by public health departments over culture tests, probably due to the delay. 1981 of course was the year that Bb, the Lyme disease agent was first isolated from ticks. (The discovery was announced in 1982).

The very first Bb strain to be identified was named "B31." It was isolated from ticks collected at Shelter Island, New York. These ticks were known to bite patients who contracted a new illness that was eventually named Lyme disease. There also happens to be a bee/flower strain of spiroplasma named "B31." This spiroplasma and another strain (B39) are associated with the lethal honey bee "May disease."[32,69,74]

According to my research, the Bb agent contains spiroplasma genes (a mutant, compound spirochete). However it is entirely possible that Bb spirochetes simply attach to the surface of a larger spirochete, like passengers on a bus in a co-infected tick. When Lyme disease patients have been treated with antibiotics that address *leptospirosis* spirochetal infections, they sometimes improve. However a smaller mycoplasma component of a spiroplasma may remain, along with antibiotic-resistant mutated spirochetes and/or other co-infections.

There are over a hundred identified spiroplasma strains including those found in ticks, bees, wasps, beetles, deerflies, fruit flies, other insects, and plants. Spiroplasmas easily acquire or delete genes to survive, and they readily mutate into new forms. There are at present over 300 identified Bb strains. Bb and spiroplasma spirochetes are found in the guts of ticks and insects including deerflies, horseflies, mosquitoes, and other species. Tick nematodes can also become infected with tiny spiroplasmas; which in turn can carry wolbachia and other symbiont infections.[65-67,73,182]

It is important to screen Bb patients for spiroplasma/mycoplasma strains. These highly evolving (pleomorphic) organisms are often antibiotic resistant or can quickly develop resistance by gene mutation. This can occur under long-term antibiotic use. Like their larger spiroplasma forms, mycoplasmas require a complex medium for growth, and are tough to detect using normal stains. The most common mycoplasmas found in tickborne infections include the following. There are many mycoplasma strains. A macrolide antibiotic, *miocamycin* is said to be useful against mycoplasmas.[199]

Mycoplasma hominis
Mycoplasma fermentens
Mycoplasma pneumonia
Mycoplasma incognitus
Mycoplasma penetrans

The most common symptoms of mycoplasma infection include joint aches (arthralgias), chronic fatigue, headaches/migraines, memory loss, sleep disorders, depression, vision problems, and nervous symptom signs. These are common symptoms with Lyme borreliosis, Morgellons, Multiple Sclerosis, Gulf War Syndrome, Chronic Fatigue Syndrome, Rheumatoid Arthritis and Fibromyalgia/Myalgic Encephalopathy patients; who may benefit from mycoplasma screening.

While Bb patients may not show evidence of mycoplasma strains during acute infection, once a few Bb spirochetes degrade (i.e. initial immune defense or after antibiotics), these smaller spiroplasmas may begin to emerge where they are detectable with laboratory tests. This may be why some Bb patients have no antibodies until weeks after infection; when spirochetes begin to break down under immune challenge. Once the (spiroplasma) outer surface proteins begin to discard, they degrade into their smaller mycoplasma forms. We tend to think of Bb as having a protein coat or envelope. However, some outer surface proteins (OSP) may simply be bacterial attachments. Unmutated spiroplasmas, Bb, and another spirochete called a *Leptospira* all cast off outer proteins to survive.[86,165]

Leptonemas

Perhaps the most important clue to tickborne illness involves a little-known bacterial spirochete called a *Leptonema.* This is a mutated form of a well-known bacterial parasite, a *Leptospira.* Leptospira spirochetes are found throughout the world. They infect insects, plants, animals, and humans (*Leptospirosis*). These spirochetes live in soil and water; especially that which is polluted. Human leptospirosis is very common around the world, and there are many different strains. Some leptospires were classified as non-infectious (saprophytes). Others were felt to be infective pathogens. However it has been concluded that even so-called non-pathogenic strains can cause infections.[134]

Many people have leptospirosis infections and are completely unaware since symptoms widely vary. Pets including cats, dogs, and horses carry and transmit leptospirosis infections through body fluids including urine, blood, semen, milk, and saliva. Animals, birds, reptiles, and insects also harbor leptospirosis infections; including more than one strain.[200]

Drinking and tap water, and all fresh and salt water sources contain leptospires since they are ubiquitous to the environment and too small for water purification. *The pollution and contamination of leptospires in the environment is a recognized public health issue.* For example, in 1998, two men were infected with leptospirosis when swimming in an Illinois lake. The CDC reported that leptospires were the cause of their infections. The agency recognized that recreational exposures to natural water sources is a common route of leptospire transmission. Indeed public health officials have been tracking leptospirosis and some mutated leptospira infections in turtles, bulls, and other animals since the 1940's.[13,16,112,113,117]

Like Bb spirochetes, leptospires have *segmented genomes* (genes) that can be swapped with other bacteria; particularly in the presence of phage viruses and DNA-disrupting chemicals or enzymes. Segmented genes are like beads on a chain. Since DNA is made up of phosphates, any phosphate-based chemicals (i.e. those used industrially or agriculturally) have the potential to disorder, break, or help to rearrange microbial genes. Remember, ticks and animals become partly infected with what lies within soil and water, including mutated or unmutated leptospires.[82,83,117,147]

In 1917 Dr. Hideyo Noguchi isolated a new kind of leptospira that was named after him (*Leptospira* Noguchi 1917). He compared it to two kinds of human spirochetes, *spironema* and *treponemes.* (The spironema were later called "borrelia." Treponemes include the syphilis spirochete, to which Bb is said to be somewhat similar). The new "Noguchi 1917" was classified as a *Leptonema* strain; or in other words a new, intermediate (mutant) spirochete. In later years, Noguchi's lonely leptonema would find company with another new leptonema strain that would be isolated from a Romanian river (1953); and then others from livestock (1965), and from a Connecticut human Lyme patient in August, 1981.[13,16,68-71,85]

The human leptonema was isolated by Connecticut Rheumatologist Allen C. Steere and his team; which they cultured from a Lyme patient's EM rash. The patient was among an early cluster of Lyme cases in the state. The patient was bitten by a tick that May. The team named the leptonema *Leptospira inadai Lyme* after a Japanese scientist (Inada) and the area where the patient lived (Old Lyme/Lyme).[13,16,68-71]

The strain was tested against a spirochete that had been isolated in 1952 from an Australian man. The strain reacted at a low titer to *Leptospira celledoni. L. celledoni* belongs to a serogroup of animal leptospires (*Leptospira borgpetersenii*). The group includes *Leptospira tarassovi*, a turtle strain. Turtles and rodents live in wet conditions where ticks thrive, including lakes, rivers, and water treatment plant ponds.

The new "*Leptospira inadai* Lyme" is from a pathogenic group of leptospires called *Leptospira inadai icterohaemorrhagiae* (serogroup Ictero). This very long name describes an animal pathogen that is part rodent (inadai), part cattle leptospire (icterohaemorrhagiae).[68-71]

However this pathogen does not address any possible spiroplasma component to a Bb organism, if it does indeed have one. You can read the important history of the odd turtle and cattle leptonema infections that were sought, found, and named by public health experts; and learn about spiroplasma history and discovery in two of my books.[13,16,69]

During the early days of the Connecticut outbreak; just like spiroplasmas, Bb spirochetes were difficult to culture, although leptospires were not. The scientists who studied Lyme in the early days did not have a sensitive enough culture medium to properly visualize spiroplasmas. Spiroplasmas and mutated leptospires may have visually looked the same under a microscope. A better culture medium was quickly developed by National Institutes of Health scientist Dr. Alan Barbour just months after the discovery of the mutated leptonema spirochete in the Lyme patient's skin. The new culture medium was used to isolate and culture the Bb agent shortly thereafter; followed by its announcement to the world.[69]

The presence of a mutated leptospire in a Lyme patient's skin rash could mean that the infection known as Lyme disease (particularly if it involves a bull's-eye rash), involves a leptonema spirochete. If so, it is multiply infected, and carries agents which vary by strain. Is a mutated leptospira/spiroplasma (leptonema) the infamous *Borrelia* (tick-transmitted agent) *burgdorferi* named after Dr. Burgdorfer?

It appears that a Lyme bull's-eye rash might have a fungus/virus/mutant bacterial spirochete as a causative agent. If nothing else, the possibility of the presence of leptonemas within Lyme patients who exhibit a bull's-eye rash deserves more than a shoulder shrug. This appears especially valid since a mutant spirochete was found in a Lyme patient's EM rash during the Connecticut outbreak; immediately before the agent of Lyme disease was suddenly discovered under a modified culture technique.

I was intrigued when I suffered from bacterial sepsis, and I was treated intravenously with a different generation of antibiotic than what is used to treat Lyme patients. The drug is Keflex, which is said to be effective when treating certain leptospirosis infections. The drug saved my life with the added benefit of a significant improvement in many Lyme symptoms. It was for this reason that I began exploring the role of leptospirosis as a possible component of Lyme disease. It was shortly thereafter that I discovered that a mutated leptospira had been cultured from a Lyme patient's skin.

I found a list of leptospirosis infection-related antibiotics in a textbook. Different strains were said to be sensitive to different antibiotics. The book was edited by a spirochaetologist who is intimately connected with Lyme disease history. The book was published following a Minnesota conference in June 1975; the year the Connecticut Lyme disease outbreak was announced. Perhaps the antibiotic I took addressed a serogroup* from which my spirochetes originated (before mutation). It would be interesting if Bb spirochetes respond by serogroup to the antibiotics that address the unmutated leptospira serogroups such as those listed in my source.[69,86]

**A serogroup is a group of bacteriae that have antigens in common. An antigen is a substance that binds to antibodies. Antigens are used in diagnostic tests to detect Bb strains in patient blood samples.*

What Lies Within

For years I have studied early literature and the patent inventions related to Bb. Leptospira strains are described for vaccine use in a patent. Their outer membrane proteins include those in the 31-36 and 41-kDa ranges. These are identical to those of Bb spirochetes. The 93-kDa leptospira protein is important for infection. A leptospira-related patent describes Bb outer membrane proteins, revealing they are similar; and they would be if Bb is a mutated leptospira (leptonema).[137-139]

A *Borrelia burgdorferi* patent describes a formula for a vaccine or a diagnostic test. It can also be used to detect microbes in soil, water, or in microbial insecticides. It can also detect microbes that are used to bio-remediate (clean up) contaminated soils or waters, for example around nuclear plants. The device can detect bacteria which include *E. coli, Bacillus subtilis* (soil bacteria related to B.t. and anthrax), *Salmonella, Serratia marcesans, Pseudomonas* species, and phage viruses.[135]

Nuclear plants can use microbial insecticides to treat incoming water flows. Their wastewaters may include some important, radiation-resistant, difficult to treat extremophile bacteria and other microbial remnants which can mutate under radiation. If any of these microbes make their way into our bodies by a tick bite, they may be difficult or impossible to kill.

The first Bb strain to be identified came from the east coast; downstream from a nuclear plant. It is also interesting that mutated leptonemas first emerged in the world in two countries downstream from where nuclear plants or nuclear machines (i.e. betatrons) were in operation.[13,16]

Another Bb patent was invented by scientists including Thomas Schwan from Hamilton, Montana (National Institute of Health's Rocky Mountain Labs). Dr. Schwan was one of the co-authors of the paper which (along with Dr. Willy Burgdorfer) announced the causative agent of Lyme disease to the world. The patent describes Bb proteins that are discarded by the body; and which can be detected using the device.[136]

The patent seeks antibodies or fragments of antibodies to a major Bb protein at 83-kDa. The 83-kDa protein is not among the antibody markers that are said to be important in the current CDC-recommended standardized Lyme disease laboratory diagnostic tests,* although it has shown up as the 83/100 (a/k/a p93) band in European strains. The patent was filed by three NIH scientists just two years before the CDC sponsored a special conference in Dearborn, Michigan where Lyme disease laboratory testing methods were formally standardized. *Pseudomonas* bacterial strains secrete infectious proteins that are detectable at 93-kDa.[136,189,190,194]

*93kDa is one of the 10 CDC bands of the IgG Western blot. If 83/100 is the 93 band, then it is included.

Dr. Schwan, one of the patent inventors, was an investigator at the Dearborn conference where he supplied Bb antibodies for the immunoblot tests used in the conference workgroup studies. The workgroup helped standardize the two-tiered diagnostic tests to detect human Lyme disease. Today these same tests are still recommended and used by many physicians on suspected Lyme patients. The patented device detects spirochetes including *soil bacteria.* It can also detect other important microbes found in tickborne infections, and in foods that have been exposed to microbial insecticides.[136,141]

The patent also detects the chemical bioremediating *Pseudomonas* strains that are found in nature, and in agricultural or industrial insecticides. Among the microbes the device is "particularly useful" for are these infections, most of which are tickborne:

- *Borrelia burgdorferi*
- Relapsing fevers (*Borrelia hermsii, B. duttoni, B. turicatae*)
- *Leptospira interrogans* (pathogenic leptospires)
- *Mycoplasma pneumonia* (remember mycoplasmas are spiroplasmas)
- *Bacillis anthracis* (anthrax, the relative of *Bacillus thuringiensis or B.t., the agricultural insecticide that is in global use*)
- *Chlamydia* species (*C. psittaci, C. trachomatis*)
- *Pseudomonas aeruginosa* (or other *Pseudomonas* species)
- *Helicobacter pylori*
- *Coxiella burnetti* (Q fever agent)
- *Francisella tulerensis* (Tularemia)
- *Rickettsia* species (*rickettsii, akari, prowazekii, tsutsugamushi*)
- *Clostridium* species (*perfringens, botulinum*)
- *Legionella pneumophila*
- *Listeria monocytogenes*
- *Neisseria* species (*meningitidis, gonorrhoeae*)
- *Campylobacter jejuni*
- *Mycobacterium* species (*tuberculosum, avium*)
- *Treponema denticola; T. pallidum* (human syphilis spirochete)
- *Bacteroides* species (*B. fragilis, B. gingivalis*) [136]

From the patent:

"The sources include but are not limited to environmental sources such as soil, water, air. The present invention allows microorganisms from water supplies, waste treatment sites, oil spills, mines, and agricultural areas to be isolated by immune capture and cultivated."

"Also of interest as a source are tissues and fluids from <u>ticks</u>, lice, reduviid bugs, mosquitoes, flies, and other vectors known or suspected of being involved in the transmission of infectious microorganisms to animals."[136]

An important Bb protein that was identified in recent years is in fact, the 93-kDa protein. In Lyme patients with chronic infections, this is sometimes the *only* diagnostic band that will show up positive on non-standardized IgM* tests. The 93 band is excluded from (CDC standardized) reportable bands for IgM Western blot tests, but it is included for the IgG Western blot. This means that 93 shows up during later infections; perhaps after Bb organisms discard some of their proteins (degrade).[137-139,191-193]

**IgM is Immunoglobulin M, the first antibody produced during Bb infection. Western blot tests for Lyme disease check for the presence of IgM and IgG antibodies. IgG is Immunoglobulin G, an abundant antibody produced during the secondary stage of infection. Antibodies may persist over time or be entirely absent in seronegative patients who are infected with Bb. Standardized laboratory tests for Lyme disease are able to detect only a fraction of Bb strains that are presently found in patients with Lyme disease. Therefore other, more specific and sensitive tests are being used. Despite the value of these tests, some public health experts will still only recommend the CDC-two-tiered test strategy to screen potential Lyme patients.*

Several patent inventions of Dr. Alan Barbour appear to hint at the connections between *Borrelia burgdorferi, Pseudomonas aeruginosa,* and *Leptospires*. (Dr. Barbour was also a Dearborn conference participant; is a borrelia patent-holder, and one of the scientists who developed the special culture medium used to isolate the Bb agent).[144-146]

One reference cited in a Barbour patent for a "flagella-less" borrelia diagnostic test is: *Loss of virulence associated with absence of flagellum in an isogenic mutant of Pseudomonas aeruginosa in the burned-mouse model*. (Montie et al. Infect. Immun. 1982;38:1296-8).

Other references cited in Barbour et al. patents refer to leptospires and to brush border membranes. The latter are gut tissues found in insects, arthropods, animals, and humans. B.t. insecticides produce holes in the brush border membranes of insects and ticks. This enables infections to enter their circulation. This release facilities the reactivation of latent and introduced infections; contributing to rapid death. Some of the references cited within these patents discuss leptospires and gut tissues:[144-146]

> *Axial filament involvement in the motility of Leptospira interrogans.* (Bromley, Charon. J Bacteriol. 1979; 137:1406-1412);
>
> *Motility of the spirochete Leptospira.* (Goldstein, Charon. Cell Motil Cytoskel. 1988; 9:101-110);
>
> *Adhesive properties of Vibrio cholerae: nature of the interaction with isolated rabbit brush border membranes and human erythrocytes.* (Jones, Freter. Infect Immun. 1976; 14:240-245).
>
> *Antigenic variation is associated with DNA rearrangements in a relapsing fever Borrelia.* (Meier et al. Cell. 1985; 41:403-9).

Note the reference to human erythrocytes (blood cells), since B.t. insecticides have been found to infect human blood cells. Also note that relapsing fever borrelia mutate. Relapsing fevers are tickborne infections. It sounds as if scientists are discussing organisms that can become part of a mutated spiroplasma/leptospira (*Leptonema*) like the one found in a Lyme patient's skin rash in 1981. Remember that discovery occurred just months before the *Borrelia burgdorfer* agent was announced to the world and named after Dr. Burgdorfer. *Is an insecticidal bacteria and a leptospira part of a mutated Bb spirochete?*[19,20,23,69,147]

Dr. Burgdorfer was studying ticks as hosts to leptospirosis infections during the late 1950's. Less than a decade later he would isolate a unique spiroplasma spirochete from rabbit ticks. In the 1950's, mutated leptonemas would be isolated from a European river. They would also be isolated from bulls at an Illinois animal research facility, and from turtles collected from Illinois and Georgia counties near rivers, ponds, and wastewater treatment plants – downstream from nuclear plants.[13,16]

Is Bb a complex mutant organism? Its bloated *genome* (collection of genes) would suggest that it is. If so, it appears to be composed in part with plant/tickborne spiroplasmas and an animal leptonema (i.e. rodents, cattle, turtles). Whatever fungi/yeast/viruses/bacteriae/parasites that a tick contracts contributes to its toxic infection payload. No wonder patients are so ill; depending upon the number and kind of microbes in an individual mutated Bb strain, which presents as a tick-transmitted *infection complex.*

We might examine the region from which the tick that bit any patient came. If we do, we may find important clues to the origins of a mutated spirochete within the individual patient's body. We may also find clues to other important, multi-layered infections that are part of the patient's tickborne illness – including those that persist despite antibiotic treatments (i.e. extremophiles).[69,81,84-85]

Three patent inventions describe the ten genetic groups of the leptospira family (*Leptospiraceae*). Please pay attention to their names (serovar means type).[148-156]

- *Leptonema illini* serovar illini (Illinois bull and turtle strains)
- *Leptospira biflexa* serovars patoc, semaranga, and codice (aquatic, so-called "non-infectious" saprophytes)
- *Leptospira interrogans* serovars icterohaemorrhagiae, fort bragg, ballum, celledoni, and borincana (animal pathogens)
- *Leptospira interrogans* serovar Lyme (A pathogenic leptospira strain classified as "Lyme")

Ten DNA samples used in these patents were supplied by the National Pig Disease Center in Ames, Iowa. Each patent describes diagnostic tests which detect the agent of swine dysentery. This is a swine (gut) enterobacteria; or what some reports label as "swine flu."[148-156]

The patents also indicate there is a pathogenic (animal) leptospira that is named "Lyme." Is this an admission that "Lyme" disease is caused by a mutated animal leptospira? Is it evidence that Lyme disease is related to the so-called "swine flu"? Could this also mean that "swine flu" vaccines might also target Lyme or leptospirosis infections?[148-156]

Is Bb an animal-derived, tick-transmitted pathogenic leptospira or leptonema like that cultured from a Connecticut Lyme patient? Is *Leptospira inadai* Lyme a mutated, aggregate leptonema that causes human Lyme disease, but that was instead renamed *"Borrelia burgdorferi"*?

Other "leptonema" patents describe leptospira outer membrane proteins. One patent makes important statements about Lyme infections about which not every public health expert admits:[152-154]

> *"Both syphilis and Lyme borreliosis are characterized by widespread dissemination early in the course of disease, including invasion of the central nervous system...Leptospira share this ability with other pathogenic spirochetes such that meningitis is a common manifestation of leptospirosis. Another feature of spirochetal infections is the ability to persist chronically in the host, as manifested in cases of tertiary Syphilis and chronic Lyme arthritis."*

The patent mentions the *persistent and chronic nature* of leptospirosis and Lyme disease infections; and the neurologic disease that can be caused by both. This would certainly make sense if Bb spirochetes are partly made of mutated leptospires.[152-154]

Tickborne infections as we can see, can have many components to them because there are many pathogens inside of ticks. This supports the idea that patients will have persistent infections that are not quickly addressed using only short-course or single dose antibiotics. They will likewise be difficult to detect using only one or two standardized laboratory tests that are limited to only one or two bacterial strains.

Since there are numerous infectious agents in any given tick's body, there is no practical way to define all tickborne infections. There certainly appears to be no logical reason to adhere to rigid published infectious disease guidelines that cannot address multi-tiered infections.

There is also no logic behind attacking physicians at the state medical licensing level for treating patients who have complex infections. Some physicians have lost their licenses or had them suspended simply because complex infections force them to use non-standardized therapies not described in a single infectious disease guidelines publication.

The CDC says that tickborne infections should be diagnosed based upon clinical symptoms and tick exposure risk. Patients should not be dismissed on the basis of a single, or two-tiered set of standardized tests that are unable to detect most strains of Lyme disease; or the many other pathogens that we now know appear on and within ticks across the globe.

Persistence Is Proven

We may now look at the larger picture of Lyme disease as a complex group of infections and parasites that are transmitted by ticks. Each patient's infection complex is therefore unique because they are not dealing with a single, but with multiple organisms. Although the core organisms are distinctively *borrelia,* their composition outside of a few key components may prove to be highly and regionally variable. Considering all the different microbes that can assemble into bacterial mutants; the number of possible Bb strains that can form, is staggering.

Physicians must consider that patients are infected with tick-transmitted fungi, viruses, bacterial mutants, parasites, and other pathogens. They must consider that the patient's immune system is also burdened with heavy metals and other toxins. These combined stressors add to the disease process. They cannot possibly be addressed by 30 days of a single antibiotic; or even a short-term series of intravenous antibiotics.

To assume that one course of antibiotics or of any treatment therapy can meaningfully address multi-tiered infections that vary between patients around the world, is illogical. Therefore, multiple therapies for longer durations for different class organisms appears to be supported by the evidence in this book, in research papers, and in the patients in the clinician's office.

Understanding that some of these pathogens are antibiotic resistant; that they may mutate, and that others may be extremely difficult to cure, further complicates the treatment approach to tickborne infections. It also underscores the need for far more flexibility in treatment, in physician "disciplinary" hearings, and in testing recommendations.

It also necessitates that public health experts globally acknowledge that tickborne infections cannot possibly adhere to strict infectious disease clinical practice guidelines currently being promoted. Guidelines are often cited by insurance companies, disability agencies, and others who lack information (such as that within this booklet), to deny benefits to patients.

In the first book of my Lyme book series *"It's All In Your Head: Patient Stories From the Front Lines,"* I discuss human transmission of

Lyme disease and other tickborne infections. Person-to-person transmissions include sexually, by body fluids (i.e. semen, saliva, milk, blood), tissue/organ transplants, and transmission in the womb.[27]

It is quite obvious that tickborne infections are transmitted through these routes, not only because there is extensive literature proving same, but because entire families are infected with tickborne illnesses. Many of these people do not recall ever having a tick bite.[13,16,27]

During my research into Bb persistence, I learned that many microorganisms use biofilms in nature to commune within for protection. The Bb spirochete, leptospires, spiroplasmas, and the bacteria *Pseudomonas aeruginosa* each form or persist within slimy biofilms. Biofilm lovers are treatment-resistant organisms.

A patent invention claims to reduce or inhibit bacterial biofilm formation. The invention describes the use of ursolic and asiatic acids; chemicals that are useful for example, in cosmetics. These acids also inhibit certain cancers (i.e. breast cancer). The invention describes a biofilm inhibitor derived from the plant *Cenella asiatica.* This is the Asian pennywort (Manimuni). It is used in Ayurvedic and traditional Chinese medicine.[157,158]

There are a number of reliable sources which describe the persistence of Lyme disease. I wish to illustrate that for many years, academic scientists have known about the chronic, serious nature of tickborne infections. However, physicians and some public health officials are not listening to patients; or researchers who are patenting products related to tickborne agents. There are many other sources proving that Lyme is complex, serious, and chronic; and that patients can be seronegative.

1.) Eight patients with skin lesions received antibiotics before study entry. One patient had a lesion for two months despite antibiotic treatment. Seven of eight study patients developed neurologic, cardiac, or joint abnormalities. – Steere AC, Malawista SE, Hardin JA, et al. Erythema chronicum migrans and Lyme arthritis. The enlarging clinical spectrum. An Inter Med 1977;86:685-698.

2.) Five patients received tetracycline in acute Lyme when they had EM rashes. All patients developed *"significant complications" despite treatment that met or exceeded "current recommendations."* – Dattwyler RJ, Halperin JJ. Failure of tetracycline therapy in early Lyme disease. Arthrit & Rheum 1987;30:448-450.

3.) Bb spirochetes were demonstrated in the brain and liver of a newborn infant whose mother had Lyme, but who had been treated with oral penicillin during her first trimester. The authors concluded that the newborn's death was likely from respiratory failure, caused by perionatal brain damage. – Weber K, Bratzke HJ, Neubert U, Wilske B, Duray PH. Borrelia burgdorferi in a newborn despite oral penicillin for Lyme borreliosis during pregnancy. Ped Infect Dis J 1988;7:286-9.

4.) The authors studied 17 acute Lyme patients who received "prompt" treatment with antibiotics. The authors noted that despite oral antibiotics, *chronic Lyme disease "subsequently developed."* This appears to be a recognition of chronic Lyme by three infectious disease doctors who co-wrote Infectious Diseases Society of America (IDSA) medical guidelines for diagnosing and treating Lyme disease. – Dattwyler RJ, Volkman DJ, Luft BJ, Halperin JJ, Thomas J, Golightly MG. Seronegative Lyme disease. Dissociation of specific T- and B-lymphocyte responses to Borrelia burgdorferi. New Engl J Med 1988;319(22):1441-6.

5.) Spirochetes and "globular antigen deposits" were detected in and around normal and injured lymph blood vessels in 6 of 12 patients. The authors commented that as in tertiary syphilis or tuberculoid leprosy, the stimulus for antigenic response in Lyme arthritis appeared to be a small number of spirochetes which, according to the authors, *"may persist in the synovial lesion for years."* The study was undertaken in part by a Connecticut Rheumatologist who has been key to Lyme disease history. – Steere AC, Duray PH, Butcher EC. Spirochetal antigens and lymphoid cell surface markers in Lyme synovium and tonsillar lymphoid tissue. Arthrit & Rheum 1988;31:487-495.

6.) Despite antibiotic treatment, post-therapy patients developed neurological symptoms such as paresis of muscles in the extremities (with radicular distribution), and cranial nerve palsies. These are considered to be symptoms of chronic Lyme neuroborreliosis. – Kohler J, Schneider H, Vogt A. High-dose intravenous penicillin G does not prevent further progression in early neurological manifestation of Lyme borreliosis. Infec 1989;17(4):216-7.

7.) The authors concluded that the persistence of Bb after antibiotics in early infection and chronic Lyme disease cannot be excluded in Bb seronegative patients. Study patients later developed Lyme disease symptoms despite antibiotic treatment. Because of this, the authors question whether a complete eradication of Bb is even possible with antibiotics. – Preac-Mursic V, Weber KL, Pfister HW, Wilske B, et al. Survival of Borrelia burgdorferi in antibiotic-treated patients with Lyme borreliosis. Infect 1989;17(6):355-9.

8.) This study's author concluded that as in other spirochetal infections, early antibiotic treatment is effective. Yet he outlined treatment problems in late Lyme disease. He stated that not all patients who manifest neurologic or arthritis symptoms will respond to oral or intravenous antibiotics. He suggested that retreatment may be appropriate in persons who relapse (i.e. recurrent arthritis). He also stated that in late Lyme disease, patients who are refractory to treatment (difficult or impossible to treat) may be found. – Schoen RT. Treatment of Lyme disease. Connecticut Med 1989;53(6):335-337.

9.) Five of seven patients studied continued to have symptoms post-treatment despite a lapse of four month's time. – Nadelman RB, Pavia CS, Magnarelli

LA, Wormser GP. Isolation of Borrelia burgdorferi from the blood of seven patients with Lyme disease. Amer J Med 1990;88:21-26.

10.) The authors suggested that clinical relapse may occur in active Lyme infection, even after antibiotics. They claim that the *"latency and relapse phenomena" suggests that spirochetes survive within the host "for prolonged periods of time."* In this study, sixteen biopsies revealed spirochetes incubated for up to 10-1/2 months. They concluded that Bb is slow to divide. They concluded that some Lyme patients may require more than 2-3 weeks of antibiotics to eliminate slow-growing strains. – MacDonald AB, Berger BW, Schwan TG. Clinical implications of delayed growth of the Lyme borreliosis spirochete, Borrelia burgdorferi. Acta Trop 1990 Dec;48(2):89-94.

11.) The authors concluded that Lyme symptoms frequently required retreatments, even in patients who already received previous therapies. The authors cited *poor clinical response in about 5% of patients, despite "longer and more frequent parenteral therapy."* – Agger W, Case KL, Bryant GL, Callister SM. Lyme disease: clinical features, classification, and epidemiology in the upper Midwest. Med (Baltimore) 1991 Mar;70(2):83-90.

12.) Of 33 patients with Lyme neuroborreliosis who were treated with IV ceftriaxone or cefotaxime for 10 days; an 8.1 month follow-up showed that in 10 of 27 patients, symptoms remained. The authors noted that borrelia persisted in the CSF of one patient. It was their conclusion that prolonged therapy may be necessary in patients with Lyme disease. – Pfister HW, Preac-Mursic V, Wilske B et al. Randomized comparison of ceftriaxone and cefotaxime in Lyme neuroborreliosis. J Infec Dis 1991 Feb;163(2):311-8.

13.) Of 32 patients with Lyme disease who came from a primary care practice, (each about 16 months post-treatment), none showed persistent or recurrent symptoms. The authors found however that ELISA and immunoblot tests *were not helpful* identifying persistence in certain Lyme patients in their study. – Feder HM Jr., Gerber MA, Luger SW, Ryan RW. Persistence of serum antibodies to Borrelia burgdorferi in patients treated for Lyme disease. Clin Infec Dis 1992 Nov;15(5):788-93.

14.) Bb was recoverable long after initial infection in antibiotic-treated patients. Bb resisted detection and eradication by host defenses and antibiotics. Human foreskin fibroblasts protected Bb from two-days of antibiotics. Bb not sequestered in fibroblasts was killed. Fibroblasts protect Bb spirochetes for up to two weeks. Eukaryotic cells provided a protective environment where long-term survival of spirochetes is possible. The authors felt that intracellular spaces are protective. Skin fibroblasts and keratinocytes are survival sites for Bb. (The first contact with spirochetes in the host is typically the skin.) – Georgilis K, Peacocke M, Klempner MS. Fibroblasts protect the Lyme disease spirochete, Borrelia burgdorferi, from ceftriaxone in vitro. J Infec Dis 1992;166(2):440-4.

15.) These authors claim that early Lyme infections could be cured by oral antibiotics, while advanced cases required intravenous antibiotics in large doses. They also determined a relapse rate of 16% in patients studied. – Zhonghua Yan Ke Za Zhi. Lyme disease in China and its ocular manifestations. [article in Chinese] Liu AN. Dept Ophthalmology, Chinese Navy Gen Hospital Beijing. 1993 Sep 29;(5):271-3.

16.) One study patient had a chronic, septic form of Lyme arthritis in the knee for seven years despite repeated antibiotics and multiple arthroscopic and open synovectomies of the joint. The authors documented Bb spirochetes in the synovium and synovial fluid in the joints using PCR analysis. – Battafarano DF, Combs JA, et al. Chronic septic arthritis caused by Borrelia burgdorferi. Clin Orthop 1993; 297:238-41.

17.) The authors called neurologic and urologic symptoms in all of their Lyme patients, *"slow to resolve."* All patients studied had protracted convalescence. The authors underscored that residual neurological problems and relapses of active Lyme are common. – Chancellor MB, McGinnis DE, et al. Urinary dysfunction in Lyme disease. J Urol 1993 Jan;149(1):26-30.

18.) This study by Connecticut Rheumatologist Dr. Allen Steere reveals an important statement that spirochetes may not always be eradicated with 30 days of oral antibiotics; and that from weeks to months later, and after a *"marked cellular and humoral immune response"* (to Bb spirochetes), patients who remain untreated often had chronic or intermittent large joint arthritis, especially in the knee over a period of several years. Patients with *"certain genetic and immune markers" will "possibly"* have persistent arthritis, even if treated with IV or oral antibiotics.

According to Dr. Steere, *"B. burgdorferi may occasionally trigger fibromyalgia,"* which he calls a *"chronic pain syndrome" that displays "diffuse joint and muscle symptoms."* Dr. Steere apparently felt that this "syndrome" did not appear to be responsive to antibiotics. This study shows Dr. Steere stating that the **Lyme disease spirochete can cause fibromyalgia.** (A disease that supposedly has no known cause, and which few people causally connect to a Bb infection). – Steere AC. Musculoskeletal manifestations of Lyme disease. Amer J Med 1994;88:4A-44S-51S.

19.) Bb persisted in patients with clinical symptoms of Lyme despite "obvious" and "adequate" antibiotic therapy. Spirochetal persistence was demonstrated in CSF, skin, iris, heart, and joint biopsies. The study authors explained persistence despite antibiotic therapy. They suggested that "atypical" forms can survive antibiotic treatment. – Mursic VP, Wanner G, Reinhardt S, et al. Formation and cultivation of Borrelia burgdorferi spheroplast L-form variants. Infect 1996;24(3):218-26.

20.) The authors reported on a fatal case of neuropsychiatric Lyme disease in a patient *demonstrated by progressive frontal lobe dementia, "and pathologically by severe subcortical degeneration."* The patient relapsed after antibiotic treatment. The authors concluded that Lyme disease must be considered in patients who present solely with psychiatric symptoms; and that prolonged antibiotic treatments may be required. – Waniek C, Proihovnik I, Kaufman MA, Dwork AJ. Rapidly progressive frontal-type dementia associated with Lyme disease. J Neuropsychiatry Clin Neurosci 1995;7(3):345-7.

Quote from this paper: *"What should be done when a patient has the typical Lyme disease history but negative serology? This is still a hot question especially in the USA. My strong opinion is that oral antibiotics should be given in such cases…Ordinary laboratory tests cannot be relied upon and the PCR is too expensive for routine use.* **When the whole picture leans towards Lyme borreliosis it is both ethically and medically right to treat."'** – Vartiovaara I. Living with Lyme. Lancet 1995;345:842-4.

Tickborne Illness is No Picnic

The evidence seems clear that tickborne infection patients suffer from complex infections which persist despite antibiotic treatments. The political climate around tickborne diseases, especially Lyme and the so-called Morgellons, remains harsh for patients and for the physicians who treat them. This makes finding a doctor, a diagnosis, or treatment, extremely difficult. Many doctors are hesitant to treat tickborne illness patients at all, because of the current climate.

I must speak out about the lack of understanding afforded to people with chronic tickborne infections. This lack of understanding contributes to denials of illness by family or friends; denials by trusted physicians; denials by employers, insurance companies, family courts and other courtrooms, by lawmakers, physician medical boards, and by federal and other disability benefit offices.

Furthering this lack of acknowledgement of the patients is the unusual "denial" by some public health experts that tickborne infections are a serious problem in all areas of the world, not just in a few pocketed areas in a handful of countries. There are places in many countries including the United States where people do not have to leave their homes in order to see ticks crawling upon their furniture, pets, or their loved ones.

It is so important with any illnesses, that people offer compassion and consideration; whether or not they believe a patient is in fact, ill. I cannot tell you how disheartening it is to know (and sometimes to have positive evidence of tickborne infections) that a patient (or you) are ill; and family members or friends remain unconvinced that what you are dealing with is real, debilitating, and often life-threatening. Imagine what it is like to be a struggling patient who is repeatedly told their illness does not exist because a few scientists cannot prove it in a laboratory using "evidence-based" techniques or mathematical algorithms.

When people have tickborne infections that are hard to detect, a common knee-jerk reaction of a physician who is pressed for time is to prescribe a pill to mask symptoms. But under treating or failing to treat tickborne infections is a serious disservice to the patient; and one which sets them up for life-long illness. Tickborne infections do kill people, and this fact is slowly making its way into the news media as if it were somehow a new finding. There is no excuse for doctors to be complacent if their patients continue to have clinical symptoms. Please consider screening patients for tickborne infections.

A refusal to treat tickborne infections beyond 30 days is not always the physicians' fault. I believe there is a lack of accurate information available to the public, to physicians, and to some public health experts. While many doctors specialize in one area of research, others specialize in another area. This and other reasons including academic research climates and patent interests prevent the free exchange of important and life-saving information. Because there are few people who are looking at the overall picture, the past and current public health conclusions that have been made about tickborne infections are at best, conservative.

There appears to be an obvious lack of communication between public health personnel, academic laboratories, and those who are educating physicians and student physicians. Patients have been working very hard over the past decades to get the attention of public health experts and their doctors. They have been insisting all along that they are chronically infected.

Many physicians are shocked when they discover how complex tickborne infections truly are. Others are surprised they have never learned much about these important infections while they were in medical school. It is understandable if a physician does not know the name of a rare infectious disease. But it is a shame that many do not know the names of, nor how to treat patients for tickborne infections, even in states where Lyme disease is very common (endemic).

Patients wonder why even in today's climate with the internet and free access to scientific texts, that there is a stark lack of information in the public arena or in the mass media to support the patient experience. Patients have been shouting loudly over decades that tickborne infections including Lyme disease and Morgellons are serious and persistent. Some physicians continue to call their patients "delusional" or "depressed" when standard laboratory tests cannot quantify infections to which patients are claiming to have been exposed; and this is unfortunate.

Patients are still waiting *years* before being accurately diagnosed for tickborne infections, including many that can be detected using specialty lab tests which some public health officials claim are "unvalidated." And yet specialized lab tests are detecting infections in patients who have otherwise failed routine, public health recommended "standardized" tests.

Some patients are unaware that they are infected; so they accept the many misdiagnoses given by well-meaning physicians. Even when presented with evidence of tickborne infections, many will stubbornly refuse to change treatments or accept a new diagnosis. Other patients have known all along that they have tickborne infections since they removed ticks from their bodies. Simply because they could not find a doctor willing to consider their tick exposure, or to understand that *Lyme disease is in their state, territory, or country,* these symptomatic patients remain untreated and now have to deal with chronic tickborne infections.

Other patients are dismayed to learn that their doctors know very little or nothing at all about how to treat tickborne infections. They may receive a standard 30 days of one oral antibiotic, but are then denied further treatment. No other illness that I know of requires infections to follow a set calendar; and yet this is common fare for tickborne infections.

It is time for academic institutions to better educate junior medical experts about global infectious diseases, even if it is not their area of specialty. Tick and insect-borne infections exist across the globe. They are commonplace, and the microbes being introduced into the environment have no predictable outcome for so-called "non-target" species including food plants, animals, and humans.

Some media sources prefer to err on the side of caution and to promote narrow tickborne illness opinions formed decades ago. These people are simply uneducated about these important infections that are devastating millions of people. The public are understandably angry, as their illnesses are ignored and they cannot afford the high costs of specialty labs and treatments for which insurance companies typically refuse to pay.

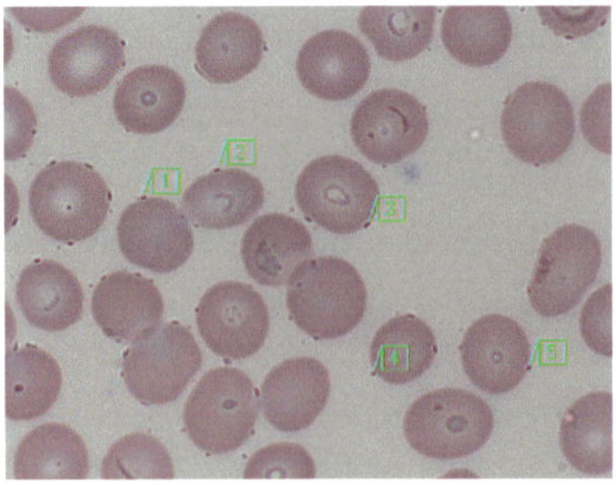

Left: A micrograph of red blood cells from a patient who is positive for *Bartonella henselae,* or cat scratch disease. Note the numbered areas where an infectious agent is adhered to the outside of the cells. Bartonella is an important *tickborne* infection. This proteobacterium is also transmitted by small animals (i.e. saliva, urine, feces). Domestic cats also carry bartonella; and toxoplasmosis, another important tickborne infection. Both are difficult to treat. In the US, approximately 90% of all domestic and feral cats are felt to have one or both of these infections. Tickborne illness patients; in particular those with anger or anxiety issues, should be screened for these often "silent" infections. Photo by the author.

As knowledge about tickborne infections has trickled forth over the past several decades, this information has not been equally shared with the public or with those responsible for creating public health policy. It is time that the truth about tickborne infections is available for all to see. It is my hope that this news will bring warring factions together so we may have a clearer view in the days ahead on how to treat very ill populations.

Tick Identification

Some people have difficulty identifying ticks. They are tiny, and many people have never seen a tick up close. The next images hint at a few common hard and soft-bodied tick species. If you would like laboratory help identifying ticks, see the list at the back of this book or check with a local public health department for instructions on specimen preservation.

Hard-shelled Ticks

(All CDC images except where marked.)

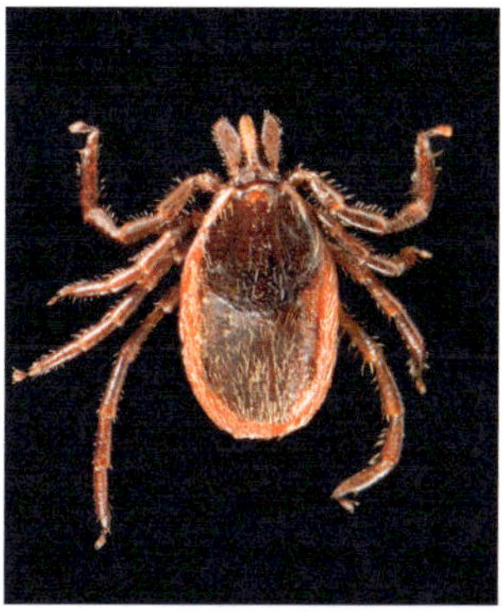

Image (right) 1975 World Health Organization (WHO).

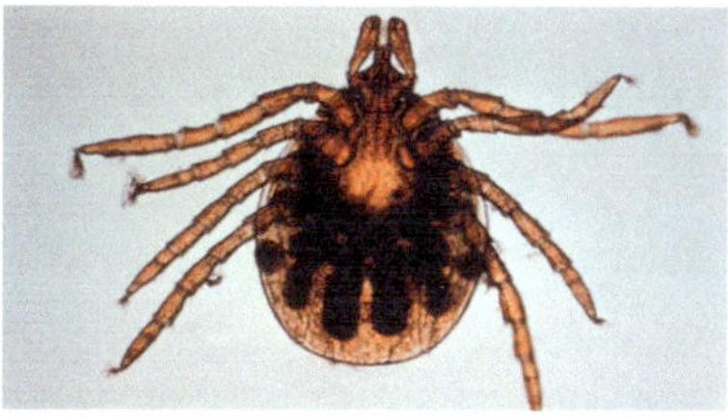

Left: *Ixodes scapularis* (female). Above: nymph of the species, that is considerably smaller in size. *Ixodes* are called "hard ticks" due to the presence of a dorsal (back) plate. There are over 200 species of *Ixodes* ticks, and many of them are able to transmit Lyme disease and other important infections.

Below: Four *Amblyomma maculatum* ticks (feed upon mammals and birds). L to R: larva, nymph, adult male, adult female. The larva is smaller than the 2mm head of a pin, and it cannot be felt or easily seen. Image CDC/Dr. Christopher Paddock.

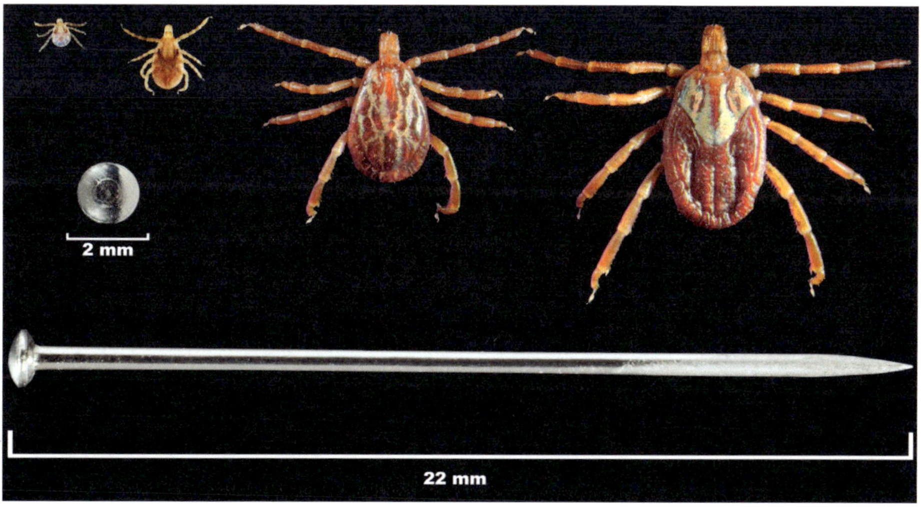

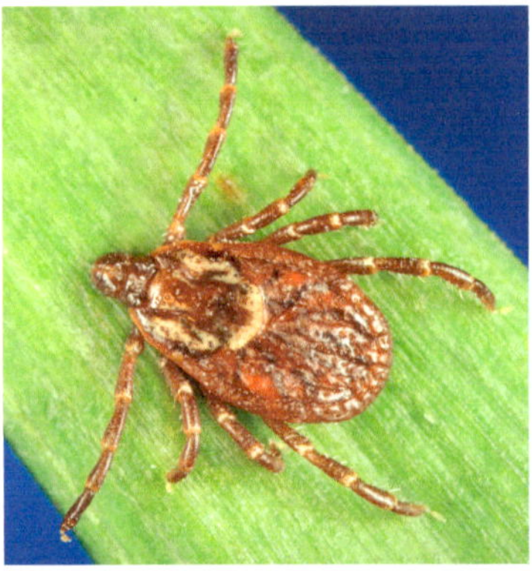

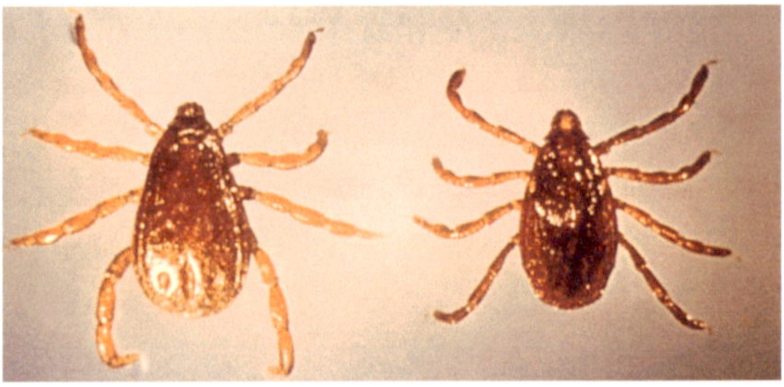

Left: Female *Dermacentor variabilis* (American dog tick). Above: Male and female *Rhipicephalus sanguineus* (brown dog ticks). Image: CDC/DVBID/Gary O. Maupin.

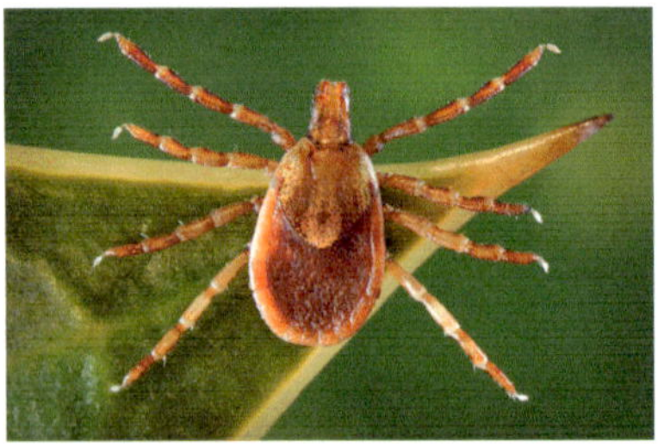

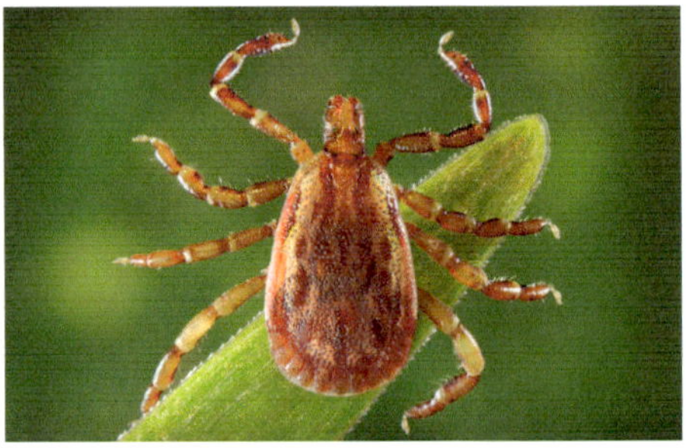

Above Left: Female *Amblyomma aureolatum* (Photo CDC/James Gathany); and Above Right: a male of the same species. (Photo CDC/Dr. Christopher Paddock.) These are yellow dog ticks, and vectors of Rocky Mountain Spotted Fever (RMSF), in Brazil.

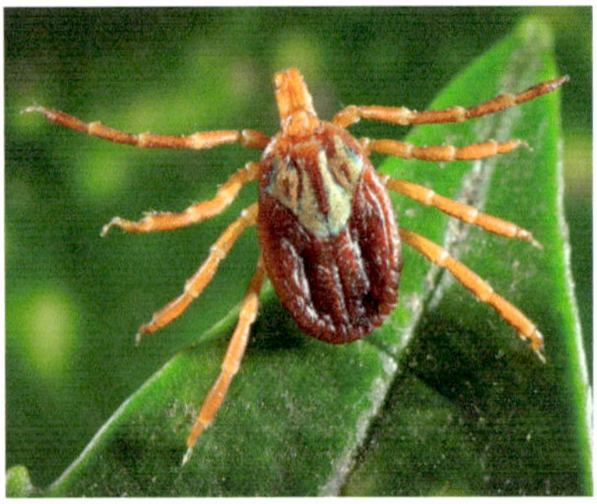

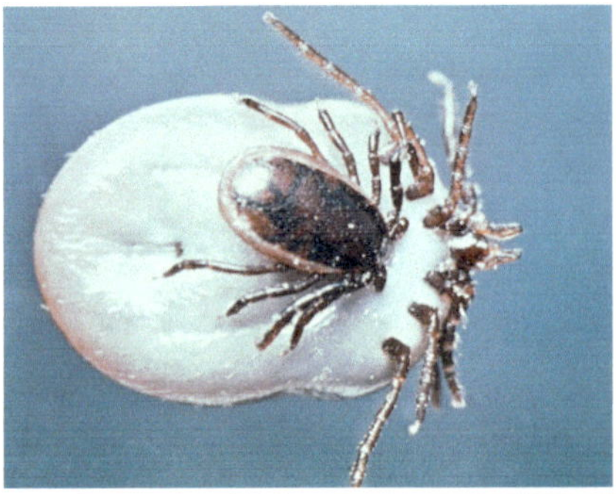

Above Left: Female *Amblyomma maculatum* (Gulf Coast tick). (Photo CDC/Dr. Christopher Paddock). Right: Male *Ixodes ricinus* (sheep) tick copulating with a female. (Image 1975 WHO).

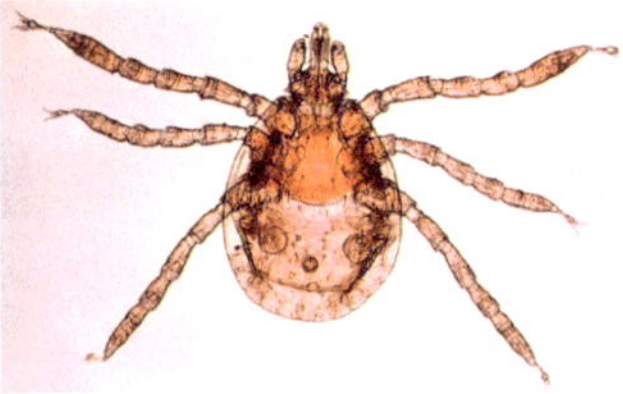

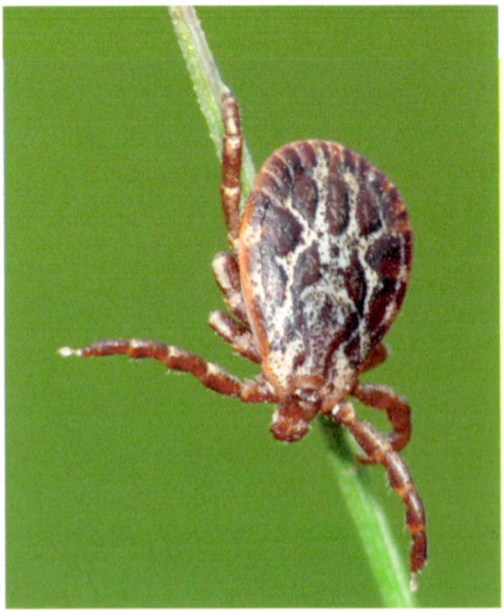

Above: Ventral (bottom) view of a larval *Dermacentor marginatus* hard tick. (Photo CDC/WHO). These ticks transmit tickborne encephalitis and Q-fever. Right: Male *Dermacentor marginatus.* Image by Lucarelli.

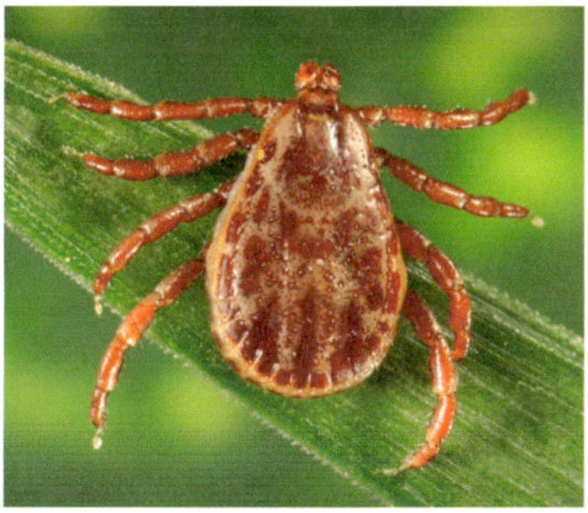

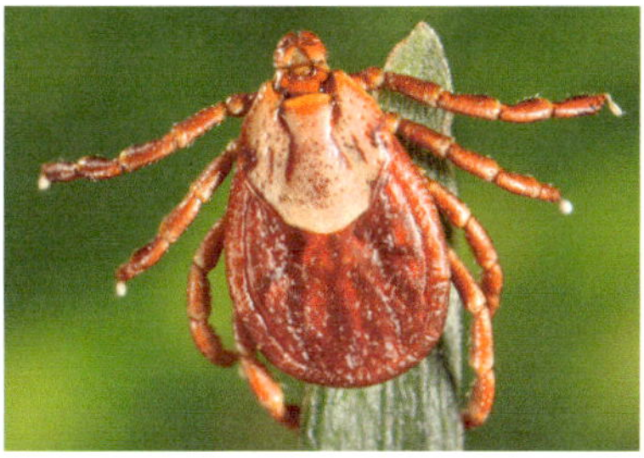

<u>Left:</u> Male *Dermacentor andersoni* (Rocky Mountain wood tick), and <u>Above right:</u> a female of the species. Photos CDC/ Dr. Christopher Paddock.

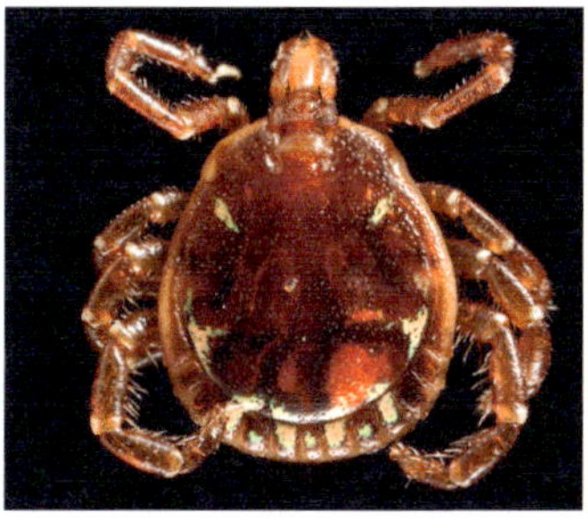

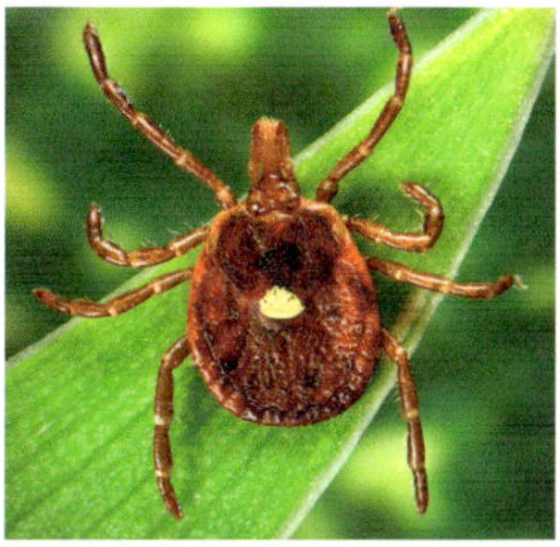

<u>Far left:</u> Male *Amblyomma americanum* (Lone Star tick), and <u>Near left:</u> a female of the species. Note distinctive "star" on the female's back. (Photos CDC/James Gathany)

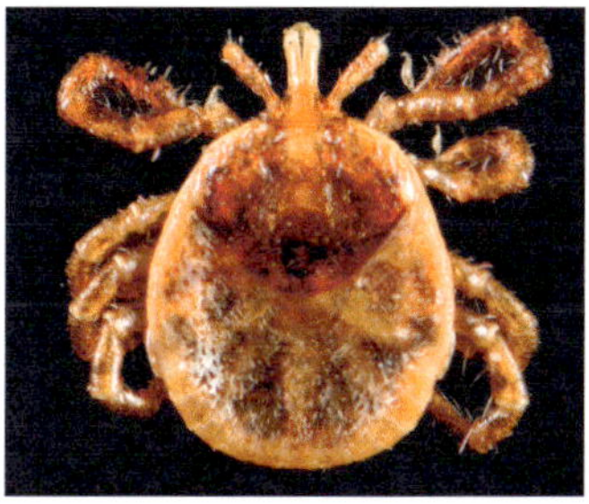

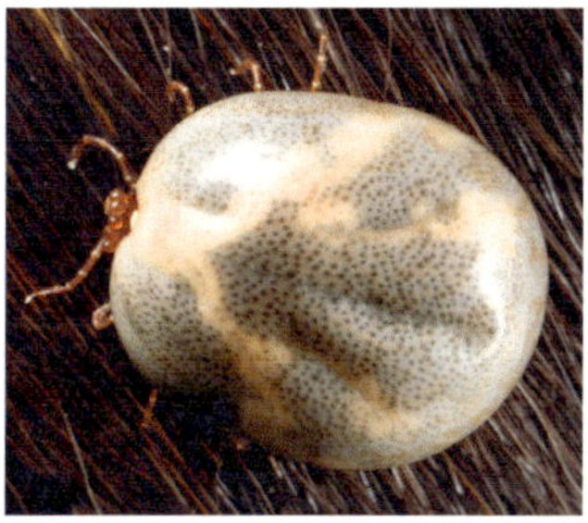

<u>Far left:</u> Immature nymph "Lone Star" tick. <u>Near left:</u> Engorged female "Lone Star" tick. Lone Star ticks transmit *Ehrlichia* and spotted fever diseases; and *Borrelia lonestari,* a Lyme-like infection that is also called Southern tick-associated rash disease (STARI). (Photos by CDC/ Drs. Amanda Loftis, William Nicholson, Will Reeves, Chris Paddock.)

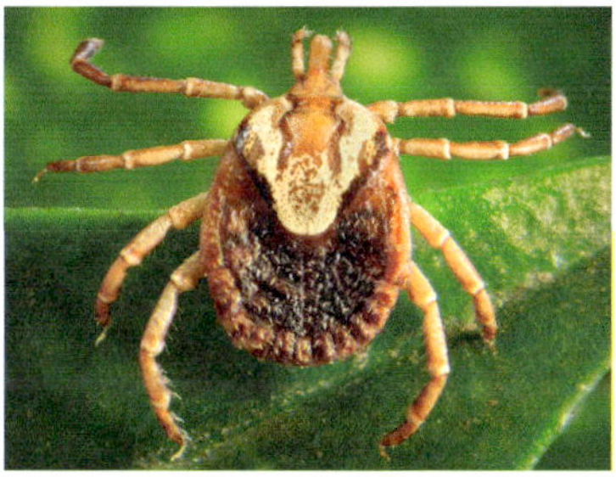

<u>Left:</u> Female *Amblyomma cajennense* (Cayenne tick). (Photo CDC/Dr. Christopher Paddock); and <u>Bottom left:</u> a male of the same species. (Photo CDC/James Gathany). <u>Below right:</u> A *Haemaphysalis* hard-bodied tick. This is a member of a peculiar group of eyeless ticks. (CDC photo).

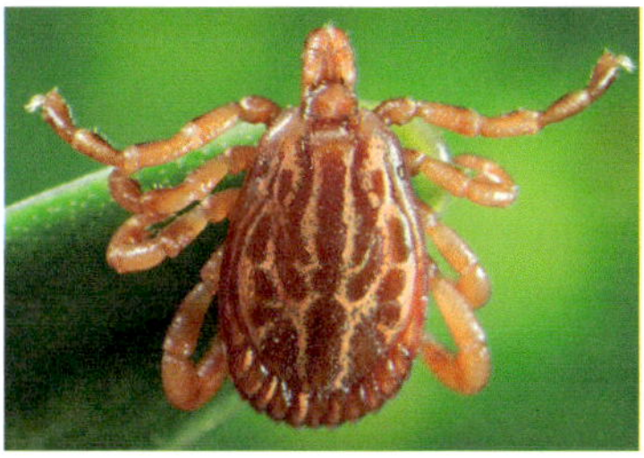

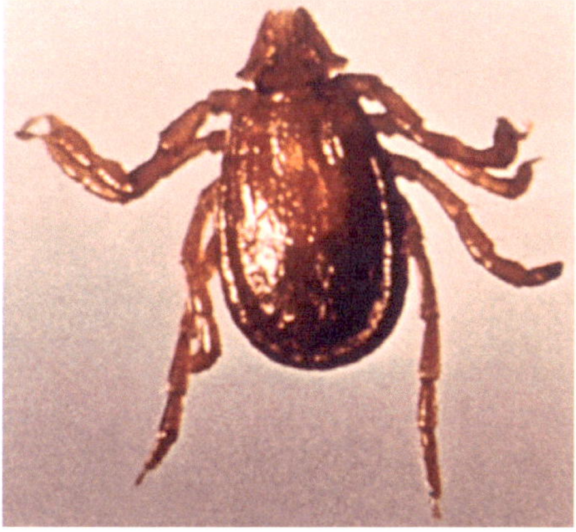

Soft-shelled Ticks

(All images courtesy of the Centers for Disease Control.)

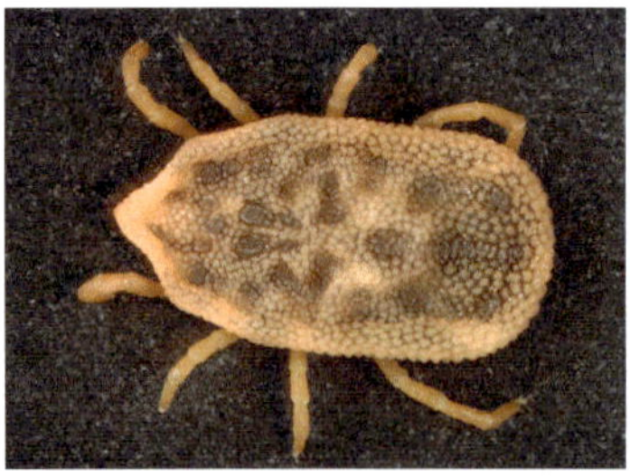

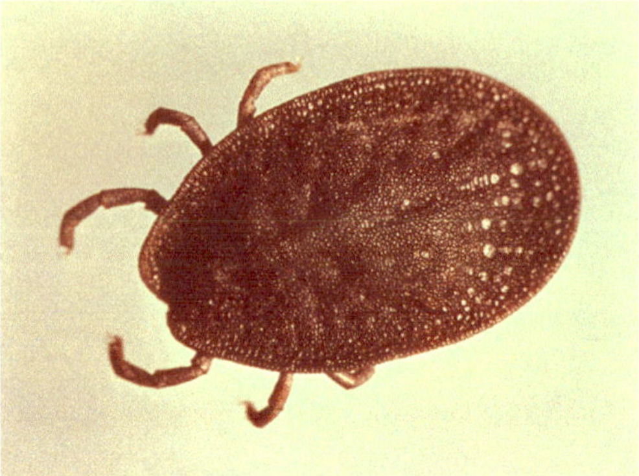

Above Left: A *Carios kelleyi,* formerly *Ornithodoros kelleyi,* or the bat tick. (Photo CDC/ William L. Nicholson, Ph.D.

Right: A member of the *Argasidae* family of North American soft ticks, and member of the genus *Argas.* This family has four groups (genera): *Argas, Ornithodoros, Antricola,* and *Otobius* ticks. (CDC image).

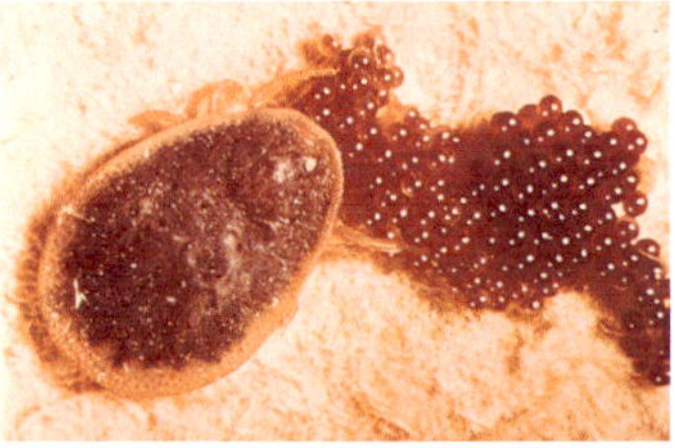

Left: A member of the *Argasidae* or soft tick family. This is a North American tick. This female has laid a batch of eggs, and over a period of several years, after each blood meal, she will lay one batch after another. Hard-shelled ticks will only lay a single batch of eggs in their lifetime.

Soft ticks are known to transmit infections called "relapsing fever" which are related to the *Borrelia burgdorferi* spirochete. Relapsing fevers produce very Lyme-like symptoms. (CDC image).

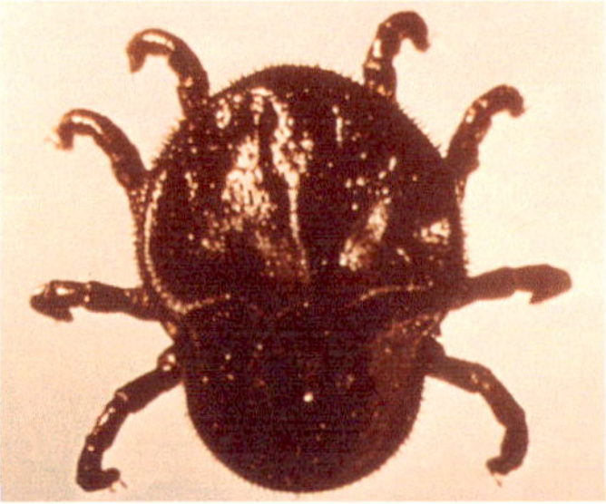

Left: A North American soft tick from the genus *Otobius.* Note its spiny body (integument). This family includes soft ear ticks. (CDC image).

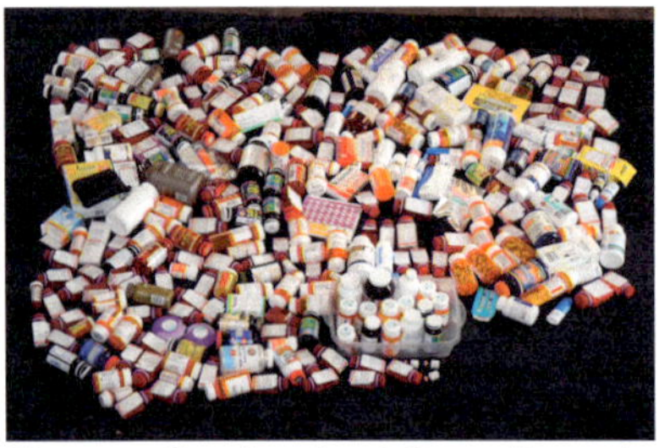

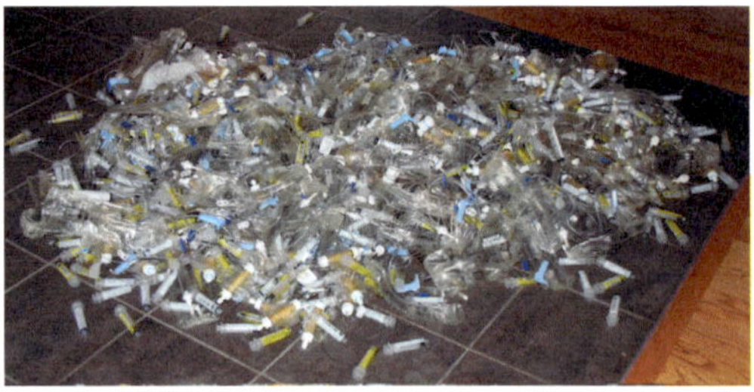

The costs of treating chronic Lyme disease that goes untreated for decades are staggering, without necessarily making the patients 100% well in all cases. Patients must be treated early and effectively as long as symptoms are present. This patient was ill for decades; had nearly 3 years of antibiotics, and is still not fully recovered. Photos Nancy Mackay.

Tick Removal and Prevention

The possibility of tickborne infections should always be taken seriously if you find a tick attached to yourself, a loved one, or your pet. It must be *properly* removed as soon as possible. The correct method of tick removal is by using a pair of tweezers or a special and inexpensive tick removal tool (i.e. tick twister) made specifically for that purpose.

Never burn a tick with a lit match or smother it in any substance. That can cause the tick to burp up the contents of its gut into your blood or to defecate on your skin. The gut, salivary glands, and excrement all contain Bb spirochetes and other important infections.

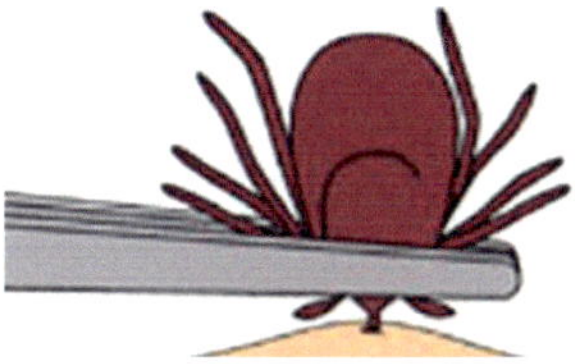

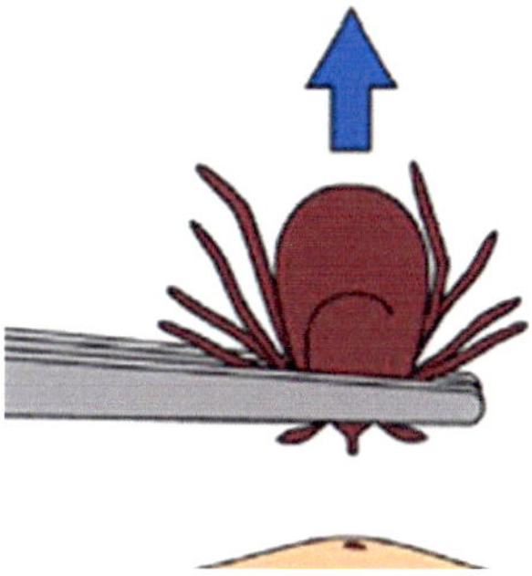

Step 1: Grasp tick firmly behind its head with tweezers.
Step 2: Pull tick gently but firmly out of the skin, ensuring that the mouth parts and head remain intact. CDC photos.

After removing the tick, disinfect the bite area. Place the tick in a plastic baggie for testing. Check with a tick testing laboratory for proper preservation techniques. Do not wait for tick testing results to return before visiting a doctor; especially if symptoms emerge.

Early diagnosis and treatment is important with all tickborne infections. If treated at onset, prognosis is good for most infections. However some may require multiple antibiotics or other supportive treatments.

If you or someone you know has been bitten by a tick, please *do not wait for symptoms to appear or assume that you are necessarily "okay."* Even if a tick was not attached for very long, they are still able to transmit many kinds of infections before, during, or upon attachment. This is because tick saliva, excrement, their mouth parts, and their bodies harbor and transmit fungi and other organisms. Ticks are also very messy eaters. They regurgitate and defecate before, during, or after their meal. This can transmit infections directly onto and into porous human skin.[165-168]

If you have had a tick attachment of any length, you may consider speaking with your healthcare provider. It is far better to be safe than sorry since ignoring tickborne infections will not make them go away.

Prevention is the Best Weapon

The best way to avoid tick-borne illness is by prevention. During outdoor travels (i.e. camping, hiking, walking, hunting), be mindful of where you walk. Ticks thrive in warmth, shade, and wet or damp environments where leaves, grass, and logs are plentiful and there is indirect sunlight. Woods, trails, farm fields, and suburban lawns are areas where ticks can be found. We do not need to be fearful of the outdoors, but we should be cautious. Here are hints to protect your family from ticks.

Before you venture out, consider some form of tick protection. Tick repellents are useful on human and pet skin (i.e. citriodiol/oil of lemon eucalyptus, rose geranium). Some products are only for clothing (i.e. DEET, pyrethrin/permethrin). Always read the label and take care, especially with children and when applying topical solutions or creams near eyes or mucous membranes.

How to Prevent Tick Bites

- Tuck pants legs into your socks before going outside. This helps to keep ticks from crawling up your pant legs.
- Choose long-sleeved, light-colored clothing; and hats or scarves to reveal crawling ticks before they attach so they may be easily removed.
- Walk in the center of paths and avoid brushing up against foliage.
- Walk pets, horseback ride, or other exercise on asphalt in tick-prone areas.
- Do not sit or lay upon leaves or grass.
- Perform frequent checks of yourself, others, and pets.
- Take turns checking for ticks, especially in hard-to-reach areas like the scalp, behind the ears, neckline, back, armpits, and behind the knees.
- When you return indoors, remove clothing and take a shower.
- Place clothing in a *hot* dryer for at least 45 minutes to kill any unseen ticks (they can easily survive a wash cycle and cooler dryer settings).
- Check pets for ticks when they come indoors, and do not sleep with pets.
- Do not allow infants to crawl upon the grass. Check diaper areas once indoors.
- Keep bird feeders away from heavily trafficked areas of the yard.
- Reduce open feeds/garbage around properties to discourage rodent infestations.
- Erect deer fences to reduce exposures to many wild animal species.

Pets and farm animals can also contract Lyme disease and other infections, and transmit them to humans. Implement landscaping techniques as a barrier between tick environments and your home (especially around ponds). Many products help reduce tick populations on deer and small animals (i.e. bait stations) and you may wish to try these products. If you find a tick, do not panic. Carefully remove it and talk to your physician.

Now that you know more about tickborne infections, you can more easily avoid them. If you become infected, this information may help your doctor to diagnose and treat you more quickly. *Enjoy the outdoors, just be cautious that you do not bring part of it home with you!*

Tick borne Infection Testing Laboratories

This list is meant to help physicians find appropriate testing for tick-borne infections. It is a list of some of the more commonly used tickborne infection testing laboratories, including those which offer specialty tests. Some of the tests offered assess the effects of tickborne infections, including hormone and endocrine imbalances, or nutritional function. It is not a complete list of labs, but it should help in the decision-making process.

North America

Advance Laboratory Services
501 Elmwood Ave.
Sharon Hill, PA 19079
Tel: 1-855-238-4949
www.advanced-lab.com/
Email contact form on site
Borrelia from culture & wellness testing

IGeneX, Inc.
795 San Antonio Rd
Palo Alto, California 94303
Tel: 1-800-832-3200
www.igenex.com
Email contact form on site
Borrelia, co-infection, tick testing

Medical Diagnostic Labs (MDL)
2439 Kuser Road
Hamilton, NJ 08690
Tel: 1-877-269-0090
www.mdlab.com
customerservice@mdlab.com
Borrelia, co-infection, other tests

Quest Diagnostics
3 Giralda Farms
Madison,NJ 07940
Main Switchboard:
Tel: 1-800-222-0446
www.questdiagnostics.com
Email contact form
Complete test list on site

Private MD Labs
Tennessee
Tel: 1-877-283-7882
www.privatemdlabs.com
info@privatemdlabs.com
Direct testing to the public

Galaxy Diagnostics, Inc.
7030 Kit Creek Rd, Ste 270
Research Triangle Park
North Carolina 27709
Tel: 919-313-9672
www.galaxydx.com
contact@galaxydx.com
Bartonella testing

Clongen
12321 Middlebrook Road, Ste 120
Germantown, MD 20874
Tel: 1-877-256-6436
www.clongen.com
akil@clongen.com
Borrelia, co-infection, tick testing

LabCorp
PO Box 2240
Burlington, NC 27216-2240
Tel: Tel: 1-800-845-6167
www.labcorp.com
Email contact form on site
Complete list on site, lab locator

Fry Laboratories, LLC
15720 N. Greenway Hayden Loop
Suite #3
Scottsdale, AZ 85260
Tel: 1-866-927-8075
www.frylabs.com
info@frylabs.com
Borrelia, co-infections incl. coccidians

R&D Systems
Minneapolis, MN (worldwide)
Tel: 1-800-343-747
Tel: 1-612-379-2956
CustomerService@RnDSystems.com
Human CXCL13/BLC/BCA-1 ELISA testing

Pharmasan Labs, Inc.
372 280th Street
Osceola, Wisconsin 54020
Tel: 715-294-1705
www.pharmasan.com
info@pharmasan.com
Complete test list on site

Spectracell Laboratories
10401 Town Park Drive
Houston, TX 77072
Tel: 1-800-227-5227
www.spectracell.com
spec1@spectracell.com
Nutritional defiiciencies, MTHFR mutation testing

Genova Diagnostics
63 Zillicoa Street
Asheville, NC 28801
Tel: 1-800-522-4762
www.gdx.net
Test list & contact form on site

Sunrise Medical Laboratories
Serving greater New York Area
Tel: 1-800-782-0282
Tel: 1-516-396-5800
www.sunriselab.com
service@sunriselab.com
Email contact form on site

South Africa

Ampath
Central Services Building
Witch Hazel Street
Highveld Office Park
Centurion (135K)
Tel: (012) 678-1001
www.ampath.co.za

Sweden

TFT-Hälsan
Mottagning i Västerås
Emausgatan 36
Tel: 021 309 309
http://tft.se/forkroppen/diagnoser/borrelia/
info@tft.se
Contact lab for testing

List Continues on Next Page

Australia
Australian Biologics Testing Services
Fayworth House, Suite 605 6th Floor
379-383 Pitt Street
Sydney, NSW 2000
Tel: +61 (2) 9283 0807
www.australianbiologics.com.au
Contact form on web site
Borrelia and co-infection testing

Germany
Infectolab
Dr. A. Schwarzbach & Dr. C. Nicolaus
Morellstraße 33
86159 Augsburg
Tel : +49 (0) 821 4550 740
www.infectolab.de
service@infectolab.de
Borrelia and comprehensive co-infection, celiac,organ profile, heavy metal testing

ANIMAL & TICK TESTING

Animal Health Diagnostic Center
Bruce Akey, MS, DVM, Director
PO Box 5786, College of Veterinary Medicine
Cornell University
Upper Tower Road
Ithaca, New York 14853-6401
Tel: 1-607-253-3900
https://ahdc.vet.cornell.edu/news/lyme.cfm
Lyme testing for dogs and horses

Analytical Services, Inc.
Attn: Tick Testing
130 Allen Brook Lane
Williston, VT 05495
Tel: 1-800-723-4432
tick@analyticalservices.com
Dry tick in ziplock bag, no alcohol or tape, Write name, address, phone, email, results 1-5 days

Connecticut Pathology Laboratories
Attn: Tick Testing
1320 Main Street, Suite 24
Willimantic, Connecticut 06226
Tel: 1-860-450-1823
Tick in damp paper towl in ziplock bag, must fill out tick testing request form available from the lab, call for form. Results 5-7 days.

Imugen, Inc.
Attn: Tick Testing
220 Norwood Park South
Norwood, Massachusetts 02062
Tel: 1-781-255-0770
Dry tick in ziplock bag. Write name, address, phone number, email on bag. Results within <10 days.

New Jersey Laboratories
Attn: Tick Testing
1110 Somerset Street
New Brunswick, New York 08901
Tel: 1-732-249-0148
Dry tick (more $ if tick is in alcohol) in ziplock bag with water-moistened cotton ball. Name, address, phone, email. Results <10 days.

Northeast Infectious Disease Diagnostic Lab
Attn: Tick Testing
314 Independence Road, Suite 114
East Stroudsburg, Pennsylvania 18301
Tel: 1-570-422-7885
Place dry tick in ziplock bag. No alcohol or tape. Must fill out tick submission form, call for form. Results <10 days.

UMass Extension Tick Assessment
Agricultural Engineering Building
250 Natural Resources Way
University of Massachusetts
Amherst, MA 01003
Tel: 1-413-545-1055
Lyme and co-infection testing on ticks. No alcohol or tape. Place dry tick in ziplock bag. Must use tick submission form, call for form. Results <10 days.

Texas Dept. of State Health Services
Attn: Zoonosis Control N MC 1956
PO Box 149347
Austin, Texas 78714-9347
Place dry tick in a zip lock bag, include contact info Must complete their submission form, call for form

IGeneX Labs ***also does tick testing, please see their listing on the previous page.***

Literature Cited

1.) Spielman, Andrew. Determinants of Infectivity of Pathogens in Vector Ticks. Harvard University, Cambridge, MA. Report XAUSAMRDC. 1990 Nov 15.

2.) Montgomery Ruth R., Stephen E. Malawista. Entry of *Borrelia burgdorferi* into Macrophages Is End-On and Leads to Degradation in Lysosomes. Infect Immun. July 1996;64(7):2867-2872.

3.) Montgomery RR, Malawista SE. Borrelia burgdorferi and the macrophage: routine annihilation but occasional haven? Parasitol Today. 1994 Apr;10(4):154-157.

4.) Montgomery RR, Nathanson MH, Malawista SE. The fate of Borrelia burgdorferi, the agent for Lyme disease, in mouse macrophages. Destruction, survival, recovery. J Immunol. 1993 Feb 1;150(3):909-915.

5.) US Patent 6,719,983. Norris et al. VMP-like sequences of pathogenic Borrelia. Filed 8/16/02. Assignee: Board of Regents, The University of Texas System (Austin, TX).

6.) US Patent 5,747,294. Flavell, et al. Compositions and methods for the prevention and diagnosis of Lyme disease. Filed 10/7/94. Assignee: Yale Univeristy (New Haven, CT).

7.) A.C. Steere. Lyme Disease. New Eng J Med. 1989;321:586-596.

8.) Rupprecht TA, Pfister HW. What are the indications for lumbar puncture in patients with Lyme disease Curr Probl Dermatol. 2009;37:200-206.

9.) Blin-Rochemaure N., Quinet B. [Should a lumbar puncture be performed in any child with acute peripheral facial palsy and clinical suspicion of Lyme borreliosis?]. [Article in French]. Arch Pediatr. 2012 Dec;19(12):1354-1361.

10.) Burrascano Jr., Joseph J. Advanced Topics in Lyme Disease. Diagnostic Hints and Treatment Guidelines for Lyme and Other Tickborne Illnesses. Sixteenth Edition. October, 2008. Available from the International Lyme and Associated Diseases Society (www.ILADS.org)

11.) Lee Mi-Sun, Su, Li, Christiani, David. MTHFR Polymorphisms and Carcinogen DNA Damage in the Lung. Epidem. 2011 Jan.;22(1):S109.

12.) Cooksey C. Health concerns of heavy metals and metalloids. Sci Prog. 2012;95(Pt 1):73-88.

13.) Langhoff, PJ. The Fourth Monkey: An Untold History of the Lyme Disease Epidemic. Allegory Press, LLC, Hustisford, Wisconsin. 2012:196. ISBN: 978-0-978-0-9833765-1-4.

14.) Kokernot RH, Calisher CH, Stannard LJ, Hayes J. Arbovirus studies in the Ohio-Mississippi Basin 1964-1967. J Trop Med Hyg. 1969;18(5):789-795.

15.) Kokernot RH. Lone Star (LS) Strain: TMA 1381. No. 239. Am J Trop Med Hyg. 1970;19(6):1151-1152.

16.) Langhoff, PJ. God Science: The Secret World of Rampant Genetics, Hidden Illness & Biotech Profiteering. 2010-2013. Allegory Press, LLC. Hustisford, Wisconsin. ISBN: 978-0-96545-7-8.

17.) Jenner W. The Medical Times and Gazette. Clinical Lectures on Diseases of the Skin. Chapter on Roseola. 1857 Jan – June;Vol. 14 (old series Vol. 35). Begins page 181. Published by John Churchill, London, England.

18.) Ellis Jodie A. Commonly Asked Questions About Btk (Bacillus thuringiensis var. kurstaki). Department of Entomology, Purdue University. http://extension.entm.purdue.edu/GM/PDF/GMquestions.pdf

19.) Poulter Sean. GM food toxins found in the blood of 93% of unborn babies. MailOnline. 2011 May 20. [internet news article] www.dailymail.co.uk/health/article-1388888/GM-food-toxins-blood-93-unborn-babies.html. Accessed 6/12/13.

20.) Sharma Dinesh C. Toxin from GM crops found in human blood: Study. India Today Group. [internet news article] http://indiatoday.intoday.in/story/toxin-from-gm-crops-found-in-human-blood/1/137728.html. Accessed 6/12/13.

21.) Founder, Sayer Ji. Green Med Info [News blog]. New Study Links GMO Food to Leukemia. 2013 May 12. http://www.greenmedinfo.com/blog/new-study-links-gmo-food-leukemia. Accessed 6/12/13.

22.) Clair E, Mesnage R, Travert C, Séralini GÉ. A glyphosate-based herbicide induces necrosis and apoptosis in mature rat testicular cells in vitro, and testosterone decrease at lower levels. Toxicol In Vitro. 2012 Mar;26(2):267-79.

23.) Arjun. Scientists Discover Bt Toxins Found In Monsanto Crops Damage Red Blood Cells. 2013 May 11. Health. [Internet News Site]. www.collective-evolution.com/2013/05/11/scientists-discover-bt-toxins-found-in-monsanto-crops-damage-red-blood-cells/. Accessed 6/12/13.

24.) Amy R. Tuininga, Jessica L. Miller, Shannon U. Morath, et al. Isolation of Entomopathogenic Fungi From Soils and Ixodes scapularis (Acari: Ixodidae) Ticks: Prevalence and Methods. J Med Entomol. 2009 May;46(3):557–565.

25.) Jay A. Yoder, Peter E. Hanson, Lawrence W. Zettler, et al. Internal and External Mycoflora of the American Dog Tick, Dermacentor variabilis (Acari: Ixodidae), and Its Ecological Implications. Appl Environ Microbiol. 2003 Aug;69(8):4994-4996.

26.) Langhoff PJ. The Baker's Dozen & the Lunatic Fringe: Has Junk Science Shifted the Lyme Disease Paradigm? 2011. Allegory Press LLC, Hustisford, WI. ISBN: 978-0-9654580-6-1.

27.) Langhoff PJ. "It's All In Your Head": Patient Stories From the Front Lines. 2007. Allegory Press LLC, Hustisford, WI. ISBN: 978-0-9654580-2-3.

28.) Langhoff PJ. The Singing Forest: A Journey Through Lyme Disease (Revisited). 2013. Allegory Press LLC, Hustisford, WI. ISBN: 978-0-9833765-4-5.

29.) Wormser GP, Dattwyler RJ, Shapiro ED, et al. The Clinical Assessment, Treatment, and Prevention of Lyme Disease, Human Granulocytic Anaplasmosis, and Babesiosis: Clinical Practice Guidelines by the Infectious Diseases Society of America. Clinical Infectious Diseases 2006;43:1089-1134.

30.) Halperin JJ, Shapiro ED, Logigian E, Belman AI, Dotevall L, Wormser GP, et al. Practice Parameter: Treatment of nervous system Lyme disease (an evidence-based review). Report of the Quality Standards Subcommittee of the American Academy of Neurology. Neurol. 2007 Jul 3;69(1):91-102. E pub 2007 May 23 ahead of print. www.aan.com/globals/axon/assets/2878.pdf. Accessed 2007 Jul 24.

31.) Burrascano Jr. J. Advanced Topics in Lyme Disease. Diagnostic Hints and Treatment Guidelines for Lyme and other Tick-borne Illnesses. 15th Ed. 2005 Sept. http://ilads.org/files/burrascano_0905.pdf. Accessed 2007 Feb. 20.

32.) Steere AC, Malawista SE, Snydman DR, Shope RE, Andiman WA, Ross MR, Steele FM. Lyme arthritis: an epidemic of oligoarticular arthritis in children and adults in three Connecticut communities. Arthritis Rheum. 1977 Jan-Feb;20(1):7-17.

33.) Aslan M, Kasapcopur O, Yasar H et al. Do infections trigger juvenile idiopathic arthritis? Rheumatol Int. 2011 Feb;31(2):215-220.

34.) Kameda G, Vieker S, Hartmann J, et al. Diastolic heart mumur, nocturnal back pain, and lumbar rigidity in a 7-year [old] girl: an unusual manifestation of lyme disease in childhood. Case Rep Pediatr. 2012;2012:976961. Epub 2012 Sep 29.

35.) Bransfield RC, Wulfman JS, Harvey WT, Usman AI. The association between tick-borne infections, Lyme borreliosis and autism spectrum disorders. Med Hypotheses. 2008;70(5):967-74. Epub 2007 Nov 5.

36.) Viader F, Poncelet AM, Chapon F, et al. [Neurologic forms of Lyme disease. 12 cases]. [Article in French]. Rev Neurol (Paris). 1989;145(5):362-368.

37.) Michel JM, Sellal F. ["Reversible" dementia in 2011]. [Article in French]. Geriatr Psychol Neuropsychiatr Vieil. 2011 Jun;9(2):211-25.

38.) Aboul-Enein F, Kristoferitsch W. Normal pressure hydrocephalus or neuroborreliosis? Wien Med Wochenschr. 2009;159(1-2):58-61.

39.) Etienne M, Carvalho P, Fauchais AL, et al. Lyme neuroborreilosis revealed as a normal pressure hydrocephalus: a cause of reversible dementia. J Am Geriatr Soc. 2003 Apr;51(4):579-80.

40.) Samimi S, Salah S, Bonicel P. [Acquired nystagmus in a 12-year-old boy as initial presentation of Lyme disease]. [Article in French]. J Fr Ophtalmol. 2011 May;34(5):325.

41.) Krejcova H, Bojar M, Jerabek J, et al. Otoneurological symptomatology in Lyme disease. Adv Otorhinolaryngol. 1988;42:210-2.

42.) Langhoff PJ. The Singing Forest: A Journey Through Lyme Disease (Revisited). 2013 Allegory Press LLC. ISBN: 978-0-9833765-4-5.

43.) Jan Bruin, Leo P.S. van der Geest (eds.) Diseases of Mites and Ticks. 2009 Springer Science + Busines Media B.V. ISBN: 978-1-4020-9694-5-2.

44.) Hermans PG, Hart CA, Trees AJ. In vitro activity of antimicrobial agents against the endosymbiont Wolbachia pipientis. J Antimicrob Chemo. 2001:47(5):659-663.

45.) Slatko Barton E, Taylor Mark J, Foster Jeremy M. The Wolbachia endosymbiont as an anti-filarial nematode target. Symbiosis. 2010;51(1):55-65.

46.) Hubálek Z. An annotated checklist of pathogenic microorganisms associated with migratory birds. J Wildl Dis. 2004 Oct;40(4):639-59.

47.) Centers for Disease Control. Lyme disease home page. http://www.cdc.gov/lyme/ Accessed 6/14/13.

48.) Par JM Dory, Chastel C, Couatarmanach A, et al. Question Étiologiques et Épidémiologiques Posées par L'érythème chronique migrant et la maladie de Lyme. A propos de 4observations réalisées au centre hospitalier regional de Rennes. [Article in French]. Bull. Soc. Path. Exot. 1985;78(3):512-525.

49.) Studahl M, Günther G, Rosengren L. Serum S-100B protein levels in patients with herpes simplex encephalitis and tick-borne encephalitis - a marker of CNS damage during the initial stage of disease. J Neurol. 2009 Apr;256(4):586-90. Epub 2009 Apr 9.

50.) Franzen-Rohl E, Larsson K, Skoog E, et al. High diagnostic yield by CSF-PCR for entero- and herpes simplex viruses and TBEV serology in adults with acute aseptic meningitis in Stockholm. Scand J Infec Dis. 2008;40(11-12):914-21.

51.) Nilsson K, Wallménius K, Påhlson C. Coinfection with Rickettsia helvetica and Herpex Simplex Virus 2 in a Young Woman with Meningoencephalitis. Case Rep Infect Dis. 2011;2011:469194. Epub 2001 Oct 19.

52.) Carle P, Laigret F, Tully JG, Bové JM. Heterogeneity of Genome Sizes within the Genus Spiroplasma. Inter J Syst Bacteriol. 1995 Jan;45(1):178-181.

53.) Tully JG, Rose DL, Yunker CE, et al. Helical mycoplasmas (spiroplasmas) in Ixodes ticks. Science 1982;212:1043-1045.

54.) Whitcomb RF The Genus Spiroplasma. Ann Rev Microbiol. 1980 Oct;34:677-704.

55.) Borde JP, Meier S, Fingerle V, et al. CXCL13 may improve diagnosis in early neuroborreliosis with atypical laboratory findings. BMC Infect Dis 2012 Dec 10;12:344. PMID: 23228054.

56.) Meraouna Amel, Cizeron-Clairac G, Le Panse R., et al. The chemokine CXCL13 is a key molecule in autoimmune myasthenia gravis. Blood. 2006 Mar 16;108:432-440.

57.) US Patent 7,629,387. Maupin et al. Compounds for pest control and methods for their use. Filed 4/13/05. Assignee: The United States of America as represented by the Secretary of Health and Human Services (Washington, DC) and the State of Oregon acting by and through the State Board of Higher Education on behalf of Oregon State University.

58.) Tully JG, Whitcomb RF, Rose DL. et al. Characterization and taxonomic status of tick spiroplasmas: a review. Yale J Biol Med. 1983 Sep-Dec;56(5-6):599-603.

59.) Henning K, Greiner-Fischer S, Hotel H, et al. Isolation of Spiroplasma sp. from an Ixodes tick. Int J Med Microbiol. 2006 May;296 Suppl. 40:157-61. Epub 2006 Mar 9.

60.) Halos L, Mavris M, Voure G, et al. Broad-range PCR-TTGE for the first-line detection of bacterial pathogen DNA in ticks. Vet Res 2006;37:245-253.

61.) Tully JG, Rose DL, Yunker CE, et al. Helical mycoplasmas (spiroplasmas) from Ixodes ticks. Science 1981;212(4498):1043-1045.

62.) Pickens EG, Gerloff RK, Burgdorfer W. Spirochete from the rabbit tick, Haemaphysalis leporispalustris (Packard). I. Isolation and preliminary characterization. J Bacteriol. 1968 Feb;95(2):291-299.

63.) Suzuki N, Supyani S, Maruyama K, Hillman BI. Complete genome sequence of Mycoreovirus-1/Cp9B21, a member of a novel genus within the family Reoviridae, isolated from the chestnut blight fungus Cryphonectria parasitica. J Gen Virol. 2004 Nov;85(Pt 11):3437-48.

64.) Burgdorfer Willy, Lackman David. Identification of the Virus of Colorado Tick Fever in Mouse Tissues by Means of Fluorescent Antibodies. J Bacteriol. 1960 Jul;80:131-6.

65.) Burgdorfer Willy, Barbour Alan G., Hayes Stanley F., Benach Jorge L., Grunwaldt Edgar, Davis Jeffrey P. Lyme Disease – A Tick-borne Spirocheosis? Science 1982 Jun;216(18):1317-1319.

66.) US Patent. 4,721,617. Johnson RC. Vaccine against Lyme disease. Filed 1986 Aug 14, published 1988 Jan 26. Assignee: Regents of the University of Minnesota (Minneapolis, MN).

67.) Jaenike J, Stahlhut JK, Boelio LM, Unckless RL. Asociation between Wolbachia and Spiroplasma within Drosophila neotestacea: an emerging sybiotic mutualism? Mol Ecol. 2010 Jan;19(2):414-425.

68.) Hovind-Hougen Kari. Leptospiraceae, a new family to include Leptospira Noguchi 1917 and Leptonema gen. nov. Int. J Syst. Bacteriol. 1979;29:245-251.

69.) Schmid George P, Steere Allen C, Kornblatt Arnold A, Kaufmann Arnold F, Moss C. Wayne, Johnson Russell C, Hovind-Hougen Kari, Brenner Don J. Newly Recognized Leptospira Series ("Leptospira inadai" serovar lyme) Isolated from Human Skin. J Clin Microbiol. 1986 Sept.;24(3):484-486.

70.) Fraser CM, Casjens S, Huang WM, et al. Genomic sequence of a Lyme disease spirochaete, Borrelia burgdorferi. Nature 1997 Dec 11;390:580-592.

71.) Noguchi Hideyo. Morphological Characteristics and Nomenclature of Leptospira (Spirochaeta) Icterohaemorrhagiae (Inada and Ito). J Exp Med. 1918;27:575-598.

72.) Brinton Lyle P., Burgdorfer Willy. Cellular and Subcellular Organization of the 277F Agent, the Spiroplasma from the Rabbit Tick *Haemaphysalis leporispalustris* (Acari: Ixodidae). Inter J Syst Bacter. 1976 Oct;26(4):554-560.

73.) Joseph G. Tully, David L. Rose, Conrad E. Yunker et al. Spiroplasrna ixodetis sp. nov., a New Species from Ixodes pacificus Ticks Collected in Oregon. Inter J Syst Bacter. 1995 Jan;45(1):23-28.

74.) Mouches C, Bové JM, Tully JG, Rose DL, McCoy RE, Carle-Junca P, Garnier M, Saillard C. Spiroplasma apis, a new species from the honey-bee Apis mellifera. Ann Microbiol (Paris). 1983 May-Jun;134A(3):383-97.

75.) Weisburg WG, Tully JG, Rose DL, et al. Source: Department of Microbiology, University of Illinois, Urbana 61801. A phylogenetic analysis of the mycoplasmas: basis for their classification. J Bacteriol. 1989 Dec;171(12):6455-67.

76.) David Taylor-Robinson, Christiane Bébéarb. Antibiotic susceptibilities of mycoplasmas and treatment of mycoplasmal infections. J Antimicrob Chemo. 1997;40:622–630.

77.) Tully JG, Rose DL, Yunker CE, Cory J, Whitcomb RF, Williamson DL. Helical mycoplasmas (spiroplasmas) from Ixodes ticks. Science. 1981 May 29;212(4498):1043-5.

78.) Stalheim OHV1, Ritchie AE1, Whitcomb RF2. Cultivation, serology, ultrastructure, and virus-like particles of spiroplasma 277F. 1USDA National Animal Disease Center (Ames, IA); 2USDA Plant Protection Institute, Agricultural Research Science and Education Administration (Beltsville, MD). Current Microbiol. 1978 Dec.;1(6):365-370.

79.) Stalheim Ole HV, Ritchie Alfred E. Whitcomb Robert F. Cultivation, Serology, Ultrastructure, and Virus-

Like Particles of Spiroplasma 277F. Curr Micrbiol. Vol. 1. 1978:365-370.

80.) Burgdorfer W, Brinton LP, Hughes LE. Isolation and characterization of symbiotes from the Rocky Mountain wood tick, Dermacentor andersoni. J Invertebr Pathol. 1973 Nov;22(3):424-34.

81.) James W. Glosser, Catherine R. Sulzer, Mark Eberhardt, William G. Winkler. Cultural and serologic evidence of Leptospira interrogans serotype Tarassovi infection in turtles. J Wildlife Dis. 1974 Oct;10:429

82.) Beaurepaire C, Chaconas G. Topology-dependent transcription in linear and circular plasmids of the segmented genome of Borrelia burgdorferi. Mol Microbiol. 2007 Jan;63(2):443-453.

83.) Beaurepaire C, Chaconas G. Topology-dependent transcription in linear and circular plasmids of the segmented genome of Borrelia burgdorferi. Mol Microbiol. 2007 Jan;63(2):443-53.

84.) Burgdorfer Willy. The Possible Role of Ticks as Vectors of Leptospirae. I. Transmission of Leptospira pomona by the Argasid Tick, Ornithodoros turicata, and the Persistance of This Organism in Its Tissues. Exper Parasitol. 1956;V:571-579.

85.) Meleney HE. Relapse Phenomena of Spironema Recurrentis. J Exp Med. 1928 Jun 30;48(1):65-82. And Berks G, Goodwin LG. Terramycin and Spironema duttoni Infections. Nature 1951 Mar 17;167(4246):447-448.

86.) Russell C. Johnson (ed). The biology of parasitic spirochetes. Academic Press Inc., New York. 1976. Proceedings of a conference held at the University of Minnesota, Minneapoils, June 2-3, 1975. ISBN: 0-12-387050-X.

87.) Schulte, Brigid. Figments of the Imagination?" Washington Post Magazine: 2008 Jan 20;pp. W10.

88.) Morgellons Research Foundation web site. www.morgellons.org and CDC. Unexplained Dermopathy (also called "Morgellons").

89.) Savely VR, Stricker RB. Morgellons disease: Analysis of a population with clinically confirmed microscopic subcutaneous fibers of unknown etiology. Clin Cosmet Investig Dermatol. 2010 May 13;3:67-78.

90.) Skinner Charles E, Emmons Chester W, Tsuchiya Henry M. Henrici's Molds, Yeasts and Actinomycetes - A Handbook for Students of Bacteriology. Second Ed. John Wiley & Sons, London. 1945.

91.) NowPublic. "Worms-Under-Skin" Disease Puzzles Scientists. 2008 May 16. [monograph on Internet]

92.) CDC. Press Briefing Transcripts. CDC to Launch Study on Unexplained Illness. 2008 Jan 16.

93.) Schoeck RJ. Sir Thomas Browne and the Republic of Letters: Introduction. Engl Lang Notes. 1982;19(4):299-312.

94.) Shaw AB. Vicary Lecture, 1977. Sir Thomas Browne: the man and the physician. Ann R Coll Surg Engl. 1978 July;60(4):336-344.

95.) Huntley Frank Livingstone. The Occasion and Date of Sir Thomas Browne's "A Letter to a Friend". Modern Philology. 1951 Feb;48(3):157-171.

96.) Peter Mayne, John S English, Edward J Kilbane, et al. Morgellons: a novel dermatological perspective as the multisystem infective disease borreliosis. F1000 Research 2013;2:118.

97.) Stricker RB, Savely VR, Zaltsman A and Citovsky V. Contribution of Agrobacterium to Morgellons Disease. 14 January 2007, SUNY findings. www.morgellons.org/suny.htm.

98.) Micah J. Benson, Jeffrey D. Gawronski, Douglas E. Eveleigh, David R. Benson. Intracellular Symbionts and Other Bacteria Associated with Deer Ticks (Ixodes scapularis) from Nantucket and Wellfleet, Cape Cod, Massachusetts. Appl Environ Microbiol. 2004;70(1):616.

99.) Windels P, De Buck S and Depicker A. Agrobacterium tumefaciens-mediated transformation: pattern of T-DNA integration into the host genome. In Agrobacterium: From Biology to Biotechnology. Tzfira T, Citovsky V. (eds.), Springer New York 2008:441-481.

100.) Gilbert GS, JL Parke, MK Clayton, J. Handelsman. Effects of an introduced bacterium on bacterial communities on roots. Ecology 1993;74(3):840-854.

101.) Snow Brook Peterson, Anne K. Dunn, Amy K. Klimowicz, et al. Peptidoglycan from Bacillus cereus Mediates Commensalism with Rhizosphere Bacteria from the Cytophaga-Flavobacterium Group. Appl Envir Microbiol. 2006 Aug;72(8):5421–5427.

102.) Holmes B. Owen RJ. Emendation of the genus Flavobacterium and the status of the genus. Developments after the 8th edition of Bergey's Manual. 1981. p. 17-26. From: H. Reichenbach and OB Weeks (ed.), The Flavobacterium-Cytophaga group. Proceedings of the International Symposium on Yellow-Pigmented Gram-Negative Bacteria of the Flavobacterium-Cytophaga Group, Braunschweig. July 8-11, 1980. Verlag Chemie, Weinheim

103.) Lewis FR. How to Collect and Process Small Polyhedral Viruses of Insects. Northeast Forest Experiment Station. Forest Research Notes. No. 109. 1960. 8 pages. By the Forest Insect Laboratory Northeastern Forest Experiment Station Forest Service, USDA New Haven, CT.

104.) Rollinson WD, Lewis FB. How to Collect and Process Large Polyhedral Viruses of Insects. In Forest Research Notes. Forest Service, USDA, Upper Darby, PA. 1962No. 130, 6 pages. By the Forest Insect Laboratory Northeastern Forest Experiment Station Forest Service, USDA New Haven,CT.

105.) Rollinson WD, Lewis FB, Waters WE. The Successful Use of a Nuclear-Polyhedrosis Virus against the Gypsy Moth. Notes. 1965. Forest Insect and Disease Laboratory Northeastern Forest Experiment

Station Forest Service, US Department of Agriculture, West Haven, Connecticut.

106.) Stallings WC, Pattridge KA, Strong RK, Ludwig ML. The structure of manganese superoxide dismutase from Thermus thermophilus HB8at 2.4-A resolution. J Biol Chem. 1985 Dec 25;260:16424-16432.

107.) Whitehouse CA, Williams LR, Austin FE. Identification of superoxide dismutase activity in Borrelia burgdorferi. J Infect Immun. 1997Nov;65(11):4865-4868.

108.) Ouyang Z, He M, Oman T, et al. A manganese transporter, BB0219 (BmtA), is required for virulence by the Lyme disease spirochete, Borrelia burgdorferi. PNAS. 20090 Mar 3;106(9):3449-3454.

109.) US Patent application 20110306917. Martin William John. Activation of the alternative cellular energy (ACE) pathway in the therapy of diseases. Filed June 9, 2010. (South Pasadena, CA).

110.) Martin WJ. Progressive medicine. Exp Mol Pathol. 2005 Jun;78(3):218-20. Epub 2005 Apr 1. Review.

111.) Crookshank Edgar M. 1890. Manual of Bacteriology. Third Edition. New York J.H. Vail & Co. 3rd Edition. H.K. Lewis, London. 1890:322-335.

112.) CDC. MMWR Update: Leptospirosis and Unexplained Acute Febrile Illness Among Athletes Participating in Triathlons – Illinois and Wisconsin. 1998;47(32):676.

113.) Jackson LA, Kaufmann AF, Adams WG, et al. Outbreak of leptospirosis associated with swimming. Pediatr Infect Dis J 1993;12:48-54.

114.) Brinton LP, Burgdorfer W. Cellular and Subcellular Organization of the 277 F Agent, a Spiroplasma from the Rabbit Tick Haemaphysalis leporispalustris (Acari: Ixodidae). Int J Syst Bacteriol. 1976 ;26 :554 -560.

115.) von der Weid I, Alviano DS, Santos AL, et al. Antimicrobial activity of Paenibacillus peoriae strain NRRL BD-62 against a broad spectrum of phytopathogenic bacteria and fungi. J Appl Microbiol. 2003;95(5):1143-51.

116.) Centers for Disease Control and Prevention. Vol 16, Number 3, March 2010 Dispatch. Paenicillus larvae Bacteremia in Injection Drug Users.

117.) Clark HF, Rorke LB. Spiroplasmas of tick origin and their pathogenicity. In The Mycoplasmas, Volume 3. Plant and Insect Mycoplasmas. Whitcomb RF, Tully JG (ed.) New York, Academic Press. 1979 :155 -174 .

118.) McWilliam Andrew. Environmental impact of Baculoviruses. 34 page report. www.fao.org/docs/eims/upload/agrotech/2003/R7299_FTR_anx3.pdf. Accessed 6/18/13.

119.) Tumilowicz Joseph J, Alexander Aaron D, Stafford Keith. On the Contamination of Leptospira Biflexa. In Vitro. 1974;10(3&4):238-242.

120.) Brendle JJ, Alexander AD. Contamination of Bacteriological Media by Leptospira biflexa. Appl Microbiol. 1974 Sept;28(3):505-506. (From Div. of Veterinary Medicine, Walter Reed Army Medical Center, Washington, DC).

121.) Sally Jo Rubin, Sidney Perlman, Herman C. Ellinghausen Jr. Isolation of Leptospira biflexa from Commercially Prepared Deionized Water Labeled “Sterile for Tissue Culture.” J Clin Microbiol. 1980 Jul;12(1):121-123. (From St. Francis Hospital and Medical Center, Hartford, CT and National Animal Disease Laboratory, Ames, Iowa.)

122.) Johnson Russell C, Harris Virginia G. Differentiation of Pathogenic and Saprophytic Leptospires. I. Growth at Low Temperatures. J Bacteriol. 1967 Jul;94(1):27-31.

123.) Vail T, Morris J, Collier SS, Mackey B. An RNA virus in Autographa californica nuclear polyhedrosis virus preparations: Incidence and influence on baculovirus activity. J Invert Pathol. 1983 Mar;41(2):171-178 .

124.) Oker-Blom Christian and Summers Max D. Expression of Sindbis Virus 26S cDNA in Spodoptera frugiperda (Sf9) Cells, Using a Baculovirus Expression Vector. J Virol. 1989 Mar;63(3):1256-1264.

125.) US Patent 5,071,748. Miller. Mixed baculovirus compositions and uses thereof. Filed 5/15/89 published 12/10/91. Assignee: Genetics Institute, Inc. (Cambridge, MA).

126.) US Patent 5,041,379 . Fraser et al. Heliothis expression systems. Filed 3/14/88 published 8/20/91. Assignee: American Biogenetic Science, Inc. (Copiague, NY).

127.) US Patent 4,870,023. Fraser et al. Recombinant baculovirus occlusion bodies in vaccines and biological insecticides. Filed 2/8/88 published 9/26/89. Assignee: American Biogenetic Sciences, Inc. (Copiague, NY).

128.) Fraser MJ, Smith GE, Summers MD. Acquisition of Host Cell DNA Sequences by Baculoviruses: Relationship between host DNA Insertions and FP Mutants of Autographa californica and Galleria mellonella Nuclear Polyhedrosis Viruses. J. Virol. 1983;47(2):287-300.

129.) US Patent 3,54 1,203. Fogle. Protected Virus Composition for Insect Control. Filed 5/8/69 published 11/17/70. Assignee: The National Cash Register Company, Dayton, OH.

130.) US Patent 5,688,764. Johnson, et al. Insecticidal peptides from spider venom. Assignee: NPS Pharmaceuticals, Inc. (Salt Lake City, UT). Filed 2/17/95 , issued 11/18/97 .

131.) US Patent 5,874,298. Johnson, et al. Insecticidal toxins from Bracon hebetor nucleic acid encoding said toxin and methods of use. Filed 2/17/95, issued 2/23/99. Assignee: NPS Pharmaceuticals, Inc. (Salt Lake City, UT).

132.) US Patent 5,688,764. Johnson, et al. Insecticidal peptides from spider venom. Filed 2/17/95, issued 11/18/97. Assignee: NPS Pharmaceuticals, Inc.

133.) US Patent 5,674,846. Johnson, et al. Insecticidal peptides from Segestria sp. spider venom. Filed 9/4/96 , issued 10/7/97. Assignee: NPS Pharmaceuticals, Inc.

134.) Kolochine-Erber B, Mailloux M. Quelque differences entre leptospires pathogens et leptospires saprophytes.Biol Med. 1963;52:496-504. [Article in French]

135.) US Patent 5,246,844. Norris, et al. Virulence associated proteins in Borrelia burgdorferi (BB). Filed 10/22 /91, published 9/21/93 . Assignee: Board of Regents, The University of Texas System (Austin, TX).

136.) US Patent 5,403,718. Dorward, et al. Methods and antibodies for the immune capture and detection of Borrelia burgdorferi. Filed 8/11/92, published 4/4/95. Inventors: David W. Dorward, Tom G. Schwan and Claude F. Garon, all of Hamilton, MT.

137.) Willy Burgdorfer. The Possible Role of Ticks as Vectors of Leptospirae. I. Transmission of Leptospira Pomona by the Argasid Tick, Ornithodoros turicata, and the Persistence of this Organism in its Tissues. Exper Parasitol. 1956:571-579.

138.) Willy Burgdorfer. The Possible Role of Ticks as Vectors of Leptospirae. II. Infection of the Ixodid Ticks, Dermacentor andersonii and Amblyomma maculatum, with Leptospira pomona. Exper Parasitol. 1959;8:502-508.

139.) Willy Burgdorfer. Artificial Feeding of Ixoded Ticks for Studies on the Transmission of Disease Agents. J Infect Dis. 1957 Jun;100(3):212-214.

140.) Burgdorfer Willy, Barbour Alan G., Hayes Stanley F., Benach Jorge L., Grunwaldt Edgar, Davis Jeffrey P. Lyme Disease – A Tick-borne Spirocheosis? Science 1982 Jun;216(18):1317-1319. Drs. Burgdorfer and Barbour were at the Rocky Mt. Lab in Hamilton, MT; Dr. Benach was at State University of New York (SUNY) Stony Brook; Dr. Grunwaldt was at Shelter Island, NY; Dr. Davis was at the Dept. of Health and Social Services, Madison, WI and is now a WI State Epidemiologist.

141.) From the Second National Conference on Serologic Diagnosis of Lyme Disease booklet published for the event. 1994 Oct 27-29 held in Dearborn, Michigan.

142.) Luft BJ, Mudri S, Jiang W, Dattwyler RJ, et al. The 93-Kilodalton Protein of Borrelia burgdorferi: an Immunodominant Protoplasmic Cylinder Antigen. Infect and Immun. 1992 Oct;60(10):4309-4321.

143.) Volkman DJ, Luft BJ, Gorevic PD, Schultz J, Padovano L. Characterization of an immunoreactive 93-kDa core protein of Borrelia burgdorferi with a human IgG monoclonal antibody. J Immunol. 1991;9(146):3177-3182.

144.) Montie TC, Doyle-Huntzinger D, Craven RC, Holder IA. Loss of Virulence Associated with Absence of Flagellum in an Isogenic Mutant of Pseudomonas aeruginosa in the Burned-Mouse Model. Infect and Immun. 1982 Dec;38(3):1296-1298.

145.) US Patent 5,436,000. Barbour, et al. Flagella-less borrelia. Filed 1/11/91, published 7/25/95. Assignee: University of Texas System (Austin, TX). Inventors: Alan G. Barbour, Virgilio Bundoc.

146.) US Patent 5,585,102. Barbour, et al., Flagella-less borrelia. Filed 9/20/93, published 12/17/96. Assignee: Board of Regents, The University of Texas System (Austin, TX). Inventors: Alan G. Barbour, Virgilio G. Bundoc, Adriadna Sadziene.

147.) Henning K, Greiner-Fischer S, Hotzel H, et al. Isolation of Spiroplasma sp. from an Ixodes tick. Int J Med Microbiol. 2006 May;296 Suppl 40:157 -61. Epub 2006 Mar 9.

148.) US Patent 5,698,394. Duhamel, et al. Nucleotide sequences and methods for detection of Serpulina hyodysenteriae. Filed 6/1/94, published 12/16/97. Assignee: Board of Regents of the University of Nebraska. This patent was filed 4 months before the Lyme disease Dearborn, MI conference to standardize laboratory testing for Lyme disease.

149.) US Patent 5,869,630. Duhamel, et al. Nucleotide sequences for detection of serpulina hyodysenteriae. Filed 10/8/96, published 2/9/99. Assignee: Board of Regents, University of Nebraska Lincoln (Lincoln, NE).

150.) US Patent 6,068,843. Duhamel, et al. Nucleotide sequences and methods for detection of Serpulina hyodysenteriae. Filed 10/2/97, published 5/30/00. Assignee: Board of Regents University of Nebraska (Lincoln, NE).

151.) LeFebvre RB, Perng GC, Johnson RC. Characterization of Borrelia burgdorferi Isolates by Restriction Endonuclease Analysis and DNA Hybridization. J Clin Microbiol.1989 Apr;27(4):636-639.

152.) US Patent 5,837,263. Haake, et a. Leptospira membrane proteins. Filed 5/19/95, published 11/17/98. Assignee: The Regents of the University of California (Oakland, CA).

153.) Glosser JW, Sulzer CR, Eberhardt M, Winkler W. Cultural and serologic evidence of Leptospira interrogans serotype tarassovi infection in turtles. J Wild Dis. 1974;10:429-435.

154.) RD Andrews, JR Reilly, DH Ferris, LE Hanson. Leptospiral Agglutinins in Sera from Southern Illinois Herpetofauna. College of Vet. Med. Univ. of IL Urbana, IL. Bulletin Wildlife Dis Assoc. 1965 Oct;1:55-59.

155.) Tripathy DN, Hanson LE. Leptospires from Water Sources at Dixon Springs Agricultural Center. J

Wildlife Dis. 1973 Jul;9:209-212.

156.) Glosser JW, Sulzer CR, Eberhardt M, Winkler W. Cultural and serologic evidence of Leptospira interrogans serotype tarassovi infection in turtles. J Wild Dis. 1974;10:429-435.

157.) Boles BR, Thoendel M, Singh PK. Rhamnolipids mediate detachment of Pseudomonas aeruginosa from biofilms. Mol Microbiol. 2005 Sept;47(5):1210-1223. [abstract]

158.) Rogers SA, Bero JD, Melander C. Chemical synthesis and biological screening of 2-aminoimidazole-based bacterial and fungal antibiofilm agents. Chembiochem. 2010 Feb 15;11(3):396-410. Chemistry, North Carolina State University, 2620 Yarborough Drive, Raleigh, NC.

159.) Steere AC, Tenney JH, Mackel DC, Snyder MJ, Polakavetz S, Dunne ME, Dixon R. Pseudomonas species bacteremia caused by contaminated normal human serum albumin. J Infect Dis. 1977 May;135(5):729-35.

160.) R.F. Whitcomb, J.G. Tully (eds). The Mycoplasmas III. Plant and Insect Mycoplasmas. Academic Press, Inc. 1979. ISBN: 0-12-078403-3.

161.) Bernard La Scola, Marie-Noëlle Mallet, Patrick A.D. Grimont, idier Raoult. Description of Afipia birgiae sp. nov. and Afipia massiliensis sp. nov. and recognition of Afipia felis genospecies A. Syst Evol Microbiol. 2002;52:1773-1782.

162.) Anja Lührmann, Karin Streker, Anja Schüttfort, et al. Afipia felis induces uptake by macrophages directly into a nonendocytic compartment. PNAS 2001 Jun 19;98(13):7271-7276.

163.) RedOrbit. New Tick Killers Avoid Widespread Spraying. 2005 Jul 30. Associated Press/AP Online. [web page]. Available at: http://www.redorbit.com/news/health/192283/new_tick_killers_avoid_widespread_spraying/index.html.

164.) Alvey S. '4-Poster' Bait Stations Reduce Deer Ticks, Disease. U.S. Army Environmental Command. Environmental Update. 2006 Fall. [web page]. Available at: http://ac.army.mil/usaec/publicaaffairs/update/fall06/fall0610.html.

165.) Barbour AG,Hayes SF. Biology of Borrelia Species. Microbiol Revs 1986 Dec;50(4):381-400.

166.) CM Shih, A Spielman. Accelerated transmission of Lyme disease spirochetes by partially fed vector ticks. J Clin Microbiol. 1993;31(11):2878.

167.) Burgdorfer W, Hayes SF, Corwin D. Pathophysiology of the Lyme disease spirochete, Borrelia burgdorferi in Ixodid ticks Rev Infect Dis 1989;11(Suppl 6):S1442-S1450.

168.) Felsenfeld Oscar. Borreliae Human Relapsing Fever and Parasite-Vector-Host Relationships. Bacteriol Rev. 1965 Mar;29(1):46-74.

169.) Hayes SF, Burgdorfer W, Barbour AG. Bacteriophage in the Ixodes dammini spirochete, etiological agent of Lyme disease. J Bacteriol. 1983;154:1436-1439.

170.) Yoshikawa, Tetsushi. Human herpesvirus 6 infection in hematopoietic stem cell transplant patients. Brit J Haematol. 2004;124(4):421-432.

171.) ATCC 58768 Mycotypha indica Kirk et Benny. Isolation: soil, India. [web page]

172.) Benny GL, et al. Observations on Thamnidiaceae (Mucorales). III. Mycotyphaceae fam. nov. and a re-evaluation of Mycotypha sensu Benny & Bemjamin illustrated by two new species. Mycotaxon 22: 119-148, 1985.

173.) ATCC 96974. Saccharomyces paradoxis Bachinskaya, teleomorph. Isolation exudate of Quercus sp., Yalta, Ukraine. [web page]

174.) Naumov GI, Naumova ES, Sniegowski PD. Differentiation of European and Far East Asian populations of Saccharomyces paradoxus by allozyme anaylsis. Int J Syst Bacteriol. 1997 Apr;47(2):341-344.

175.) Naumov ES, Naumov GI, Molina EI. Genetic variation among European stranis of Saccharomyces paradoxus: results from DNA fingerprinting. Syst Appl Microbiol. 2000 Apr;23(1):86-92.

176.) Chatonnet Pascal, Fleury Antoine Boutou Stéphane. Identification of a New Sources of Contamination of Quercus sp. Oak Wood by 2,4,6,-Trichloroanisole and Its Impact on the Contamination of Barrel-Aged Wines. J Agric. Food Chem. 2010;58(19):10528-10538.

177.) Zygomycetes. Mycotypha. Mycotypha Fenner, 1932. [web site]

178.) Delgado-Àvila AE, Urdaneta LM, García y Albino U, et al. Mycotypha indica P.M. Kirk & Benny, in turkey dung, a new record for Venezuela. Multiciencias. 2007;7(2):176-180.

179.) Rexrode Charles O, Brown Daniel. USDA Forest Service. Forest Insect & Disease Leaflet. Oak Wilt. [web page]

180.) French DW, Stienstra WC. Oak wilt. University of Minnesota Agricultural Extension Service. Minneapolis, MN. 1980. Folder 310:11.

181.) Hillman BI, Supyani S, Kondo H, Suzuki N. A reovirus of the fungus Cryphonectria parasitica that is infectious as particles and related to the coltivirus genus of animal pathogens. J Virol. 2004 Jan;78(2):892-8.

182.) Mello AF, Yokomi RK, Melcher U, Chen JC, Wayadande AC, Fletcher J. Genetic diversity of Spiroplasma citri strains from different regions, hosts, and isolation dates. Phytopathology. 2008 Sep;98(9):960-8.

183.) European Patent Search. Patent EP0522560. Livey I, Dorner F. Method and composition for the prevention of Lyme disease. Filed 07/09/92, publication date: 12/20/06. Assignee: Baxter Aktiengesellschaft. Access: www.freepatentsonline.com/EP0522560.html.

184.) US Patent 5,466,577. Weisburg. Nucleic acid probes for the detection of Lyme disease spirochetes. Filed 10/27/93, published 11/14/95. Inventor: William G. Weisburg (Milford, MA); Assignee: Amoco Corp.

185.) US Patent 4,888,276. Shelburne. Method and composition for the diagnosis of Lyme disease. Filed 6/26/86 published 12/19/89. Assignee: Minnesota Mining and Manufacturing Company (St. Paul, MN).

186.) US Patent 3,607,235. Duncan et al. Rapid bacteriological metal extraction method. Filed 2/23/68 published 9/21/71. Assignee: British Columbia Research Council (Vancouver, British Columbia, CA).

187.) Hernandez G, Fardeau ML, Cayol JL, et al. Clostridium thiosulfatireducens sp. nov., a proteolytic, thiosulfate- and sulfur-reducing bacterium isolated from an upflow anaerobic sludge blanket (UASB) reactor. IJSEM 2002 Sept;52(5):1461-1468.

188.) Geuenich HH, Müller HE. [Occurrence of Pseudomonas aeruginosa in waste water and its behavior under biological treatment]. [Article in German]. Zentralbl Bakteriol Mikrobiol Hyg B. 1984 Jun;179(3):259-65.

189.) Spencer RC. Bacillus anthracis. Review. J Clin Pathol. 2003;56:182-187.

190.) Ulrike Hauser, Lehnert G, Lobentanzer R, Wilske B. Interpretation Criteria for Standardized Western Blots for Three European Species of Borrelia burgdorferi Sensu Lato. J Clin Microbiol. 1997 Jun;35(6):1433-1444.

191.) Laure Béven, Duret Sybille, Batailler Brigitte, et al. The Repetitive Domain of ScARP3d Triggers Entry of Spiroplasma citri into Cultured Cells of the Vector Circulifer haematoceps. PLoS ONE. 20127(10): e48606. doi:10.1371/journal.pone.0048606.

192.) Nathalie Berho, Sybille Duret, Jean-Luc Danet, Joël Renaudin. Plasmid pSci6 from Spiroplasma citri GII-3 confers insect transmissibility to the non-transmissible strain S. citri 44. Microbiol. 2006 Sept;152(9):2703-16.

193.) Nabil Killiny, Brigitte Batailler, Xavier Foissac and Colette Saillard. Identification of a Spiroplasma citri hydrophilic protein associated with insect transmissibility. Microbiol. 2006 Apr;152(4):1221-30.

194.) Bleves S, Viarre V, Salacha R, et al. Protein secretion systems in Pseudomonas aeruginosa: A wealth of pathogenic weapons. Int J Med Microbiol. 2010 Dec;300(8):534-43.

195.) US Patent Application 20090324638. Live bacterial vaccine. Dattwyler Raymond J, et al. Filed 6/12/06, published 12/31/09. Inventors: Raymond J. Dattwyler (East Setauket, NY), Maria C. Gomes-Solecki (Memphis, TN), Jozef FML Seegers (Leiden, NL). Assignee: Biopeptides Corp., New York, NY.

196.) Richard S. Ostfeld, Amber Price, Victoria L. Hornbostel, et al. Controlling Ticks and Tick-borne Zoonoses with Biological and Chemical Agents BioScience. 2006 May;56(5)383-394.

197.) Coyle David R, Murphy Matthew W, Paskewitz Susan M. et al. Belowground herbivory in red pine stands initiates a cascade that increases abundance of Lyme disease vectors. For Ecol Man. 2013;302:354-362.

198.) Cornelle University Cooperative Ext. of Suffolk County. Horticulture Diagnostic Laboratory. The Japanese Black Pine - What's Happening? 4 pages.

199.) Furneri PM, Tempera G, Bisignano G, et al. Anti-mycoplasmal activity of a new macrolide: miocamycin. Chemioterapia. 1987 Oct;6(5):341-345.

200.) Johnson RC. Leptospira. (ed) In: Baron S, (ed). Medical Microbiology. 4th edition. Galveston (TX): University of Texas Medical Branch at Galveston; 1996. Chapter 35.

Made in United States
Cleveland, OH
05 November 2026

47649163R00045